DOLYCWRT
The Days of a Country Doctor's Surgery

ROGER G. K. PENN

Dolycwrt

THE DAYS OF A
COUNTRY DOCTOR'S SURGERY

Gomer

Published in 2011 by Gomer Press,
Llandysul, Ceredigion SA44 4JL.

ISBN 978-1-84851-426-3

Copyright©Roger G. K. Penn, 2011
The Author has asserted his moral right under the Copyright and
Patents Act, 1988 to be identified as the author of the work.

Printed and bound in Wales at
Gomer Press, Llandysul, Ceredigion.

This work is dedicated
to my father and mother,
the late Dr and Mrs George Penn of Whitland

Contents

Thanks and Acknowledgements

WITHOUT THE SUPPORT of so many people, this book could not have been produced. I am genuinely grateful to everyone concerned, starting with my wife, Celeste, for all her loving help and patience.

I would like to express my sincere appreciation and thanks to the management and staff of Carmarthenshire Archives Service. John Davies, David Cooke, Terry Wells and David (Harry) Jones have been a source of great help to me during many visits to their beautiful premises, where I have enjoyed my research work. In acknowledging the extracts from *The Welshman* and the *Carmarthen Journal*, I would like to add that the essential details of the earlier years of my story would not have been possible without the availability of these delightful newspaper records from the past.

The staff of the Ceredigion Archives Service, and the Carmarthen, Haverfordwest and Merthyr Tydfil Libraries – as well as various Registry Offices across Wales – have all been very supportive. I would like to pass on my sincere thanks to everyone.

I am very grateful to Luca Dussin, an Information Assistant at the Royal College of Physicians, London, and his colleagues for providing me with an outline of the doctors' careers from the *Medical Directories*; indeed these records later shaped the story. I am also grateful for the information provided to me by the Worshipful Society of Apothecaries, the Royal College of Surgeons of both London and

Edinburgh, the Royal College of Physicians of Ireland, and the Pharmaceutical Society of Great Britain.

I would like to thank everyone who kindly gave their time to be interviewed by me, and whose contributions breathe life into this story. Likewise, I am grateful to those who provided a photograph, especially Whitland's retired photographer, Mr Rainbow of Cwmfelin Boeth and Carmarthenshire Museums Service.

It has been a privilege for me to get to know two gracious ladies, whose sharp memories have shed light onto the darkness of years gone by. I refer to Caroline Rees-Davies, the daughter of Dr Vaughan Bowen-Jones, formerly of Glan-yr-Afon, Llanboidy – who can recall spending time with Mrs Creswick Williams, the widow of the first doctor at Dolycwrt – and Nancy Davies of Tŷ Newydd, Cwmfelin Boeth, who remembers being treated as a patient by Dr Owen.

I would like to thank Dr Malcolm Holding and Dr Roy Allen, formerly of Dolycwrt Surgery, for their contributions, and also Dr David Jenkins of Ferryside, and Dr Alun Hughes, of Cwmbran, for sharing some of their reflections with me. My late father's records and speeches have also been an inspiration and, as always, I owe so much to him.

I wish to thank William Gibbon, of Pwllywhead farm, and Maurice Dunbar, of Snowdrop Cottage, for their interest and support in the project since its early beginning. I am also grateful to John Davies of Whitland, the Reverend Kingsley Taylor, John Dyer, Kenneth Kendall, Derrick Burnell, John Gibbin and Beverley Graves, as well as Keith Thomas, Clive Evans, Mair (Kirk) Thomas, and Lawrie Bowen of Whitland's former Creamery, which was Dolycwrt's next door neighbour for many years.

I have been fascinated to read the Log Books of my former school, Whitland Primary, and I would like to thank Mrs

Humphries, Head Teacher, for her kindness in arranging this. I have also appreciated being given the Minute Books of both the Whitland Memorial Hall and Whitland Week committees to read – whilst also being provided with information by the Whitland and Llanboidy Branch of the Royal British Legion.

Since I started my writing in January 2010, my work has been checked by the Writers Bureau of Manchester. I would like to thank my tutor, Penny Legg, for keeping me on track at all times, and also the Director of Studies, Diana Nadin, and her colleagues, for an excellent working relationship. May I congratulate them, too, for turning another small-time writer into a published author.

It is my pleasure to thank the good people of Whitland and its community for showing interest in my project – indeed it is our project – and for sharing their recollections of the town's former days. Many of you are mentioned in the story, but for those who are not, please be assured that I am sincerely grateful to you all.

And finally, a few words of appreciation are due to Dylan Williams, Head of Publishing at Gomer Press, and his colleagues. From the very outset, I have wanted to share this story with everyone and they have granted me this privilege. Diolch yn fawr am gymryd diddordeb yn y stori ac am y cymorth parod a roddwyd i mi.

Now, I simply invite you all to read on. I sincerely hope that this little story appeals to your fascination as it has app-ealed to mine, thoroughly, in the course of its preparation.

Many thanks, and best wishes.

ROGER PENN
Dolycwrt, 2011

Foreword

I AM DELIGHTED to say a few words about Roger's story as I am one of the fortunate few to have known most of the doctors mentioned in this book. Dolycwrt has such fond memories for me; it was a place where I was so well and kindly treated over the years.

During the past twelve months, Roger has shared his writing with me, often visiting Tŷ Newydd to read aloud his latest lines. This is a wonderful work, a fascinating and pleasant read, and a treasure for today's Whitland.

Roger links Dolycwrt's first doctor to its last, early traditional days to the later modern world – while connecting tales and events of the intervening years with a rich and golden thread.

This book will be enjoyed by anyone wishing to visit or revisit the glory days of Whitland, and by others wishing to explore life during this particular period of time. But throughout all, Dolycwrt takes centre stage – our little surgery with a big heart.

NANCY DAVIES
Tŷ Newydd, 2011

Preface

DOLYCWRT was a country doctor's surgery for exactly 100 years, beginning in 1898, when doctors opened certain rooms of their residences to patients for treatment, and ending shortly after 1998, by which time purpose-built modern health centres had been established across the country. During Dolycwrt's 100 year term, medicine experienced its greatest breakthroughs and reforms and, at the very midpoint in 1948, Wales' own Aneurin Bevan introduced the National Health Service.

This story describes Dolycwrt's remarkable journey from early humble beginnings, in late Victorian times, into a new world significantly changed by two World Wars and considerable progress in most walks of life. It reflects upon many of Whitland's former days, including Sir Winston Churchill's visit in 1941, and describes the warmth and memories of this delightful medical fortress in the heart of West Wales.

More importantly, it serves to remind us about Dolycwrt's wonderful doctors and their devotion to duty. Their unfailing efforts, expertise and caring ways earned them universal love and respect from patients in every corner of this country practice and beyond.

The story of Dr George Penn's retirement from general practice after serving at Dolycwrt for 42 years was the subject of an award-winning BBC documentary, 'The Doctor's Story', in 1998 – part of a series commemorating the 50th anniversary of the National Health Service.

Dr Creswick Williams and
the Potential of Prospect House

ON THURSDAY November 10th 1898, Dr John Thomas Creswick Williams LRCP (Lond), MRCS (Eng), LSA became the first medical man to take ownership of Whitland's modern and desirable property, Prospect House. This commanding building of great character and charm, stood tall, strong and steadfast, and the beautiful hand-cut stonework shaped its rugged looks. It had a courtyard for the carriages; a stable for the horses; outbuildings and enclosures, and a garden which extended, as a small meadow, to the bank of the River Gronw. Dr Creswick Williams had secured all of this on a long term lease for the sum of £395.

For many people, it would be the perfect residence and the perfect retreat, where, within the privacy and peacefulness of its cosy interior walls, the home fires would burn with a special red glow. For Dr Creswick Williams, however, this was to be more than a home. His proud profession had, by now, shaped a rewarding future for the hardworking General Practitioners, who welcomed the sick and poorly into their homes for treatment. Dr Creswick Williams would be no different. He recognised the potential of his new stronghold in serving others – while providing permanence for his future studies and discoveries in medicine.

At this moment in time, Whitland was a progressive little town – situated at the scene of important past history, where the rich remains of Roman times left a clear reminder of another age. In the more recent 10th century, according to tradition, Hywel Dda, 'King of all Wales,' gathered representatives of his kingdom to Whitland's same location to codify the Welsh laws.[1] The Cistercian Abbey then followed two centuries later, experiencing both peaceful monastic life and fierce battles, whilst its early-day infirmary saw to the needs of the sick and infirm. But it was hundreds of years later – long after the Abbey Ironworks had come and gone[2]– that Whitland, the small town, started to develop in early 1854. The South Wales Railway had just arrived, passing beyond the hamlets and small thatched cottages of this borderland valley, having extended its course from Carmarthen to Haverfordwest, towards the deep waters of the Haven, at Neyland.[3]

Whitland's setting, in rich green pastureland, provided farming, but it was the railways in those glorious days of steam that brought employment. Initially a small station, it grew to become an important junction point, connecting the Neyland and Milford Haven lines, and the Tenby-Pembroke service, to Carmarthen and eastern locations – and, likewise, the stations in North Pembrokeshire and Fishguard, too.[4] The Whitland and Taf Valley Railway was another busy line, linking Whitland to the slate quarry at Glogue and also the silver and lead mine near Llanfyrnach.[5] This became known as the Cardi Bach line – an affectionate description, meaning a small-time railway extending to Cardigan.

Each of the railways combined to put Whitland firmly on the map – with stores, shops, pubs and hotels soon following. Churches and chapels occupied key locations within the

---

1 *Hywel Dda Garden and Interpretive Centre, Whitland* – official leaflet.

2 *The History of Whitland*, by the Reverend William Thomas. English Translations by Ivor Griffiths.

3 *The Pembroke and Tenby Railway*, by J. P. Morris, Laidlaw – Burgess.

4 *The Railways of Pembrokeshire*, by Richard Parker ISBN 978-1-906419-07-3

5 Llanfyrnach Mine Pembrokeshire: website as at March 1st 2011.

town, all towering figures just like their respected ministers. They welcomed everyone on the Sabbath day for fellowship and thanksgiving, binding everyone together in an atmosphere of true community spirit.

In 1875, the Llanboidy and Llangan United District Board School was built, signifying the growing importance of the small town. Around this time William Henry Morgan Yelverton Esquire, of Whitland Abbey, was making plots available to purchasers as part of his generous contribution towards Whitland's development. It was on one of these plots – across the dusty road from the new school – that Prospect House was built. An extract from the original lease, dated October 7th 1881, provides a description and summary of its intended use – before it later became a surgery, known as Dolycwrt:

> All that piece of ground forming part of the field known as Parc Rhydycwrt in the parish of Llangan: bounded on the north by a garden in the occupation of William Thomas, minister of the gospel; in the south by ground in the occupation of Thomas Williams, coach builder; on the east by the river; and on the west, or front side, by the New Road (later named St Mary's Street).
>
> The Lessee will, at his own expense, within one year of the date hereof, erect to the satisfaction of the architect, a good and substantial dwelling house, with sufficient outbuildings and conveniences.

Since arriving in Whitland in 1891, Dr Creswick Williams had noticed the town's increasing activity. Each day the steam trains that regularly puffed their way into its station provided regular routines and functions, giving a sense of practical importance and belief to the small town. Dr Creswick Williams knew that the railways also had a big bearing on his professional work. With hundreds of men employed as drivers, firemen, guards, porters, shunters, engineers and others working as gang members servicing the lines, accidents could – and would – occur.

Purpose prevailed in all quarters, with passengers, journey-men, and wagon loads of goods all destined to be relocated. Travelling merchants were engaged in trade, as was Medical Hall, the small, but busy, chemist shop in St John Street. Likewise, a cobbler, blacksmiths, sawyers, wheelwrights, tailors and others plied their skills in and around the town.

Dr Creswick Williams had played a big part in this growing community. For the past seven years this physician and General Practitioner had served as the, more affectionately termed, 'Family Doctor' – as well as being the Medical Officer for Health, covering a wide area. This pivotal role in society linked him closely to his patients, whose illnesses he treated in the full knowledge of their background circumstances. Dr Creswick Williams knew that from a medical perspective he could not be nearer the source of sickness – and he was seen by everyone as a man of great importance and standing.

Residing at the stately Tŷ Gwyn ar Daf premises (meaning a White House on the river Taf – but not to be confused with 'The Old White House' of previous centuries), Whitland had become his home. Now, committing his name to the deeds of Prospect House, he was cementing his foothold. During his life, he had moved location often, but, now settled, he was enjoying this last full chapter of his medical life. It had been a most fulfilling and distinguished career for Whitland's popu-lar doctor, which had brought him travel, variety, recognition and respect – all for the price of his unfailing devotion to duty.

Early Life and The Road To West Wales

I T WAS IN THE shadow of the sharp and rugged mountains of north west Wales that Dr Creswick Williams' life began. Dolgellau, a Welsh-speaking market town, sitting beneath Cader Idris, Snowdonia, celebrated his birth in the summer of 1856. He was the son of John Williams, a local attorney's clerk, and his wife, Mary. Early family life at Smithfield Street was shared with his parents, two brothers, their servant helper, and an older gentleman who had accepted their board and lodge.[6] Slowly but surely, improved and regular schooling had become available to the young children of his age and, at least, the dreadful demands made upon working children had now been eased.

Times, however, were still extremely harsh and difficult; life was a big struggle. Many people were malnourished and poorly, and there were threats of tuberculosis, influenza and various dangerous epidemics, such as measles and scarlet fever. The generally poor and crammed living conditions – often cold, wet and damp in the winter months – brought misery to many, while the medical care available was mostly for those who could afford it.

As a growing boy, with the Grammar School only a short walk away, Creswick Williams had made up his mind to master reading, writing and arithmetic and all important subjects that followed. He looked beyond the nearby gold mines – which produced jewellery for Royal occasions – and

---

6 British Census of 1861, Meirionnydd Record Office, Dolgellau.

the important slate works, which brought time-honoured industry to this quiet, scenic corner of Wales. He was an academic, able to find his way into and around text books, and beyond examinations. More importantly, he had recognized hardship and suffering all around and this was implanted in his mind: school friends ill or dying of diseases; grown men grinding away at laborious work; everyday accidents; squalid shelter; stunted progress; limited food, and little rest.

The young Creswick Williams had read about medicine's steady advancements over the years, knowing that the genuine efforts of many ordinary people had made a big difference. England's William Harvey, explaining the circulatory nature of blood flow, was one of these – as was Edward Jenner, answering the dreaded smallpox with vaccinations. They, like so many others, were to save many lives: all alert, ambitious and determined to help human suffering. Creswick Williams recognized that proud medical schools, surgical colleges, advanced pharmacy and royal charters had now given medicine a sense of real direction. Students lay ready and waiting to explore new opportunities and, with ever-improving communications, the following century would be different. Raising his head above the parapet, he set out on the medical trail.

Creswick Williams was welcomed into the Pharmaceutical Society of Great Britain in 1877. At that time, the Lambeth district – now the home of British Pharmacy – was continuing to influence this great profession by producing various designs of colourful jars, known as delftware. Creswick Williams soon became an expert with the pestle and mortar, and, adapting well to studies in his first year, he entered the prestigious competition offered for the best herbarium. The collection of phanerogamous plants and ferns had to be presented and supported by notes in accordance with stringent guidelines, and he was to win the coveted Silver [1ˢᵗ] Prize.

In an extract from the *Pharmaceutical Journal and Transactions*, dated October 6ᵗʰ 1877 entitled 'The Botanical Prize', it was stated that Professor Bentley, when speaking about the herbarium competition, had attached great importance to botany believing:

> this science had a home amongst the students of Pharmacy, who knew its value in the future practice of their calling.

Regarding the competition that particular year, the article continued:

> There were three very meritorious collections sent in. Professor Bentley had examined them with great pleasure, especially the one to which the Silver medal had been awarded, consisting of 715 specimens . . .

This was Creswick Williams' submission, gathered in the early morning hours. It was a good start for the aspiring student, who completed his studies a few years later. Then, having registered as a 'Chemist and Druggist' in April 1879 when living at Walworth Road, Surrey, he took the next step forward.[7]

After enrolling as a medical student,[8] Creswick Williams moved to a totally different setting – the big and open valley lying to the south of Merthyr Tydfil, where large scale coal mining and iron ore extraction was taking place. At the time, the Plymouth Ironworks, situated on a site leased from the 4ᵗʰ Earl of Plymouth, was coming to the end of its considerable production life.[9] Nearby, the rich beds of quality coal were

7 The Royal Pharmaceutical Society of Great Britain.
8 Worshipful Society of Apothecaries of London, Archives Department.
9 'The Plymouth Ironworks' by Margaret Stewart Taylor M.A., F.L.A. as per the Glamorgan History, Volume 5, 1968.

being mined, and, with men and their families having moved into the area in their masses, Merthyr's population had risen enormously. Workmen's terraced houses were extending in long rows up and down the hills and valleys, where there was a need for strong medical representation for the people of this hard working community.

Moving into the nearby village of Pentrebach, situated directly behind the very grand ironmaster's house on the edge of the Works, Creswick Williams found lodgings with a working family. There, at Church Terrace, he teamed up with two young parents, Mr and Mrs Stedman, their six children and Mrs Stedman's mother. In the 1881 Census, he is described as being a 'Medical Assistant, Associate of the Pharmaceutical Society of Great Britain', and aged twenty four.[10] He was, in fact, assisting the appointed Surgeon of the Works – a seemingly endless challenge for them both, in this harsh industrial scene, at times of awful epidemic, when life expectancy was cruelly short. This would have been an eye-opening experience, and whatever he saw during his two years at the Plymouth Ironworks, when the large blast furnaces raged in the black dusty air of the crowded pits, stirred his heart and hardened his resolve.

Now with qualifications in pharmacy and invaluable medical experience, Creswick Williams satisfied all entry requirements to the famous London Hospital, taking his place as a medical student in 1882. He had earlier acquired a testimonial of his character from another medical associate, Dr Pugh MRCS, LSA, and his studies were certified by Mr Munro Scott, Warden of London Hospital and Medical College.[11] His years of dedicated study at this grand

---

10 Merthyr Tydfil Library and Archives Service.
11 The Worshipful Society of Apothecaries of London, Archives Department.

establishment fully prepared him for working life. Burning the midnight oil in paperwork was only a part of it, of course; using his scalpel in the operating theatre brought the further intensive demands of full concentration. Taking his place at the stately wards – where alcohol was then prescribed as a medicine and where the matrons ruled with an iron will – completed his education.

To obtain his surgery qualifications, he attended the Royal College of Surgeons at Lincoln's Inn Fields, London. Creswick Williams would have appreciated this fine building, with a grand entrance and portico, complete with stately columns and railings.[12] Inside, behind the old library, the exacting demands of rigorous examination awaited him. Likewise, to become Licentiate of the Worshipful Society of Apothecaries, he made an appearance at the historic Apothecaries Hall, Blackfriars, London, a city-centre location near St. Paul's Cathedral. When he arrived, he would have entered three historic and magnificent rooms – the Great Hall, the Court Room, and the Parlour – to be tested by a Court of Examiners. By obtaining all three prime qualifications, LRCP; MRCS and LSA he had become a thoroughly qualified medical practitioner.

Carmarthen's lowland location in fertile farming country-side had, by the 1880s, influenced its rise to become one of Wales' largest towns. It was there that the County Infirmary in Priory Street – the leading medical establishment in the area – set high standards in patient care. At this well respected institution, fully documented in *A History of The County Infirmary Carmarthen 1847–1948* by John Bolwell and Andrea Evans, Dr Creswick Williams had heard that a resident house surgeon's position was available. Such a post was ideal for

---

12 Personal visit to the premises by the Author.

him, and he satisfied all requirements – being unmarried, a Welsh speaker, an MRCS, and a recognised apothecary. This was to be a very prestigious role lasting three years, in a county town that cried out for professional medical care. It involved working closely with staff and patients, and his many duties included compiling a complete annual summary of accidents, operations, surgery and medical cases that were attended to during the year.

Upon leaving the County Infirmary, Dr Creswick Williams knew that he was expected to move away from the district of Carmarthen for a period of two years, so that he could not take away work from the local medical practitioners. Aberaman, a thriving coal mining village, within touching distance of the popular town of Aberdare, offered him an opening. There he practised alongside a more senior practitioner, Dr J. Bowen James MRCS (Eng) LSA, who was the listed surgeon for various coal mines and working-men's clubs.[13] This often meant that a portion of the men's wages was deducted by the mining company to pay the doctor, who would care for their families, too.

Living near to the colliery was essential. Miners, cold, wet, filthy and exhausted after a long, hard shift, would stagger home on a howling winter's night to families, often weak and poorly themselves. Difficult living conditions led to sickness, and sicknesses to epidemics. These times brought struggles for everyone including the doctors. Dr Creswick Williams and his senior partner could experience accidents and emergencies at any hour of the day. And they would set off into the grime and smog, sometimes deep-down into the bowels of the earth, with their hard-earned experience and, no doubt, their personal hopes and prayers, too.

13 The Royal College of Physicians Information Centre. *The Medical Directory.*

Entering the Taf Valley
and into the Unknown

A T THE END of his busy two years in Aberaman, Dr Creswick Williams returned to Carmarthenshire: this time deep into the county as far as its western border, where he was to settle for twenty years in Whitland. Now experienced, highly recommended and with a career path on the ascendancy, he could allow himself the comforts of a first class carriage on the Great Western steam train that chugged its way into, and out of, the many delightful small stations on the way. At this time of rigid class distinction, doctors defied the rule, being elevated somewhere above the upper class – or so it seemed. They were respected, trusted and often loved to such an extent that patients gladly opened up their hearts to them, and accepted their every word with blind faith.

As a strong Welshman, he loved the open countryside, the sea and the mountains of Wales – as well as its native tongue – and the district of Whitland provided all of these. Exciting days lay ahead. He needed his own horse and cart, and a coachman to take him down the distant country lanes. He also needed a general male servant to feed and bed his horse, and a housemaid for his food and linen. He looked forward to supporting the churches and chapels and local activities, as well as meeting the gentry of the town. Above all, he wanted to serve people to the limits of his considerable ability, with the honour bestowed upon him by the medical profession.

By the time his train left behind the quaint platform of

St Clears station, and entered into the Taf valley, the noisy braking process would signal the train's arrival on the platform edge. There would have been a welcome reception for Dr Creswick Williams that day.

He had come to assist Dr John Phillips MRCS (Eng), LSA, a more senior doctor, who had recently moved from Narberth to his grand, newly-built, home Tŷ Gwyn ar Daf, in Whitland.[14] Dr Phillips was a kind, family man, with a terrific appetite for work. Indeed he needed this. He served the Local Government Board in presiding over the medical issues of a huge area, with responsibilities, also, at the local workhouse, administered by the Narberth Poor Law Union. Now he was looking for help. Dr Creswick Williams would be the perfect assistant. He would give his heart and soul. Indeed, he knew no other way, and he would be taken into residence on the family estate.

As the Christmas of 1891 approached, the town and district suddenly fell into mourning. Dr Phillips had died, aged just 45. His health had deteriorated and Dr Creswick Williams had cared for him until the end. A peaceful sadness descended upon the Whitland valley and beyond, for Dr Phillips had been very popular and would be dearly missed. Now, only a few months into his stay in Whitland, Dr Creswick Williams' medical future had become uncertain. It was Christmas Eve, and, instead of sharing a glass of good cheer in front of a warm log fire with his new colleague, he took his place in a huge crowd of saddened figures at Soar Cemetery.[15] That dark December, the usual Christmas festivities were drowned by sorrow and shock; for Whitland and district, the new year would bring a new medical appointment.

14 *The Welshman*, 26 December, 1891, Carmarthenshire Archives Service.
15 The *Carmarthen Journal*, 1 January, 1892, Carmarthenshire Archives Service.

At that time, the events leading up to the selection of Dr Phillips' successor captured the attention of most people. Doctors were like politicians then, and people awaited this type of news with more interest than a Cabinet reshuffle. The papers provided the details and, inevitably, with more than one candidate, there would be a contest to report. There were two strong runners: Dr Creswick Williams and Dr Rowland Lewis Thomas LSA, of Henllan Amgoed, but known as Dr Rowley Thomas.

In the locality, Dr Thomas was well known and popular. And he had many interests being a lover of all aspects of country life and a keen sportsman. At rugby, cricket, billiards, whatever sport, he excelled; by nature, he was competitive, and winning came easily for him. Dr Thomas had, so far, carried-out his medical training in London, and had experience of general practice and surgery. Like his friend, Dr Creswick Williams – who was not known to have such distractions – he, too, had attended the funeral, and it was these two 'heavyweights' who contested the new vacancy, as advertised in *The Welshman* on January 9th 1892:

NARBERTH UNION

APPOINTMENT OF MEDICAL OFFICER

Notice is hereby given that the Board of Guardians will on Monday 18th January 1892 proceed to elect a Medical Officer for District No. 4, comprising the parishes of Castell Dwyran, Cyffig, Cilmaenllwyd, Eglwysfair-a-Churig, Eglwys Cummin, Henllan Amgoed, Llanfallteg East, Llanfallteg West, Llanboidy, Llanglydwen, Llangan East, Llangan West, Marros and Pendine . . . with an area of about 39,588 acres and a population, according to the local census of 4,848.

The article stated that the salary was £35 per annum, with extra income allowable for surgery, midwifery, vaccinations and other services. The elected doctor would also become Medical Officer for Health, an appointment that generated an additional salary of £20 per annum. Candidates would have to satisfy the Local Government Board with qualifications, and be knowledgeable in Welsh.

Both men had good records for looking after the poor, and this was important. 'A private patient could go to another doctor,' said one of those present at the election, 'but the poor must wait for the one appointed by the Guardians.'[16] Both men had in recent times, but for different reasons, received glowing mentions in *The Welshman*. Dr Thomas, a big community man, regularly featured in the local news. As the local contender, many in attendance that day knew him well, and were prepared to give him their vote. Indeed, one of the Guardians stated: 'As a rule, poor people liked those who had been brought up in their neighbourhood much better than those who had not.' The Chairman, however, sensing an undercurrent favouring the local candidate – duly confirmed by a petition from the local people – wanted to give Dr Creswick Williams his fair chance, and took pains to make his point, as this extract from *The Welshman* of January 23rd 1892, confirms:

> The Chairman said he would like to add that sometime ago *The Welshman* spoke in very high terms indeed of Mr Williams. He was then giving up his appointment at the Infirmary, and he (the chairman) believed the inhabitants entertained Mr Williams, or made him a presentation. It was owing to his having read those terms, and owing to the experience that Mr Williams had acquired in a colliery district, that he (the chairman) was induced to give Mr Williams his vote.

16 *The Welshman*, 23 January, 1892, Carmarthenshire Archives Service.

The ratepayers had sent the Guardians there to consider the interests of the poor, and to get for them the best medical attendance they could. If the Guardians had a local man they would not look at his qualifications so much as his being a local man. Still, it seemed to him that the Guardians ought to leave personal feelings out of the matter, and consider the interests of the poor only.

This was a close contest: now it was down to the wire; the testimonials would count. Again Dr Rowley Thomas' case was strong; there were no weaknesses in his armour. He was a competitor. He did not enter the fray to come second. No, he put his name forward to win. But then came something special. Sir Morell Mackenzie, MD physician to the late Emperor of Germany, wrote:

> I have much pleasure in stating that Dr Creswick Williams fully availed himself of the opportunities offered him at the London Hospital of obtaining a thorough knowledge of his profession. He has since acquired a very large experience and he would be a very valuable officer to the Narberth Union or any institution.

This appeared to be something of a winning shot, but only the judges would decide. Indeed, no less than forty-six Guardians – each representing their local parish – had crowded into the Board Room that day, defining this moment in local medical history. One of those was Mr W. H. M. Yelverton of Whitland Abbey, who, alongside his colleagues, now eagerly awaited the outcome. 'The vote is even, gentlemen,' declared the Chairman, to a now astonished audience. 'I give my casting vote in favour of . . .'

Dr Creswick Williams was called into the room – and the chairman continued his address:

Mr Williams, you have been elected medical officer in the place of the late Mr Phillips. You have, no doubt, heard that you saved the election by the skin of your teeth (laughter). There is no doubt about that. I feel perfectly sure that those gentlemen who have not voted in your favour will welcome you as medical officer of this board (applause); and I only trust that in the performance of your duty you will merit the confidence that has been placed in you by those who voted in your favour (applause).

A delighted Dr Creswick Williams responded:

I beg to thank you all for having elected me to the office. I feel the honour the more because I am comparatively a stranger in the neighbourhood. I know the contest has been a very keen one. Mr Thomas and I have been old friends, and I am only sorry in one way that he has lost it. As far as we are personally concerned, I think the contest has been carried on with the best of feelings. I thank those gentlemen who have voted for me, and hope to give you all satisfaction by endeavouring to do my best both for you and the paupers (applause).

No one could have doubted the responsibilities that would now rest on the shoulders of Dr Creswick Williams, or the extent of the geographical area involved. As medical officer, he was expected to promote ever-improving standards of health in his district, in every respect. This would range from encouraging people to open their windows for ventilation, to public hygiene hazards such as poor drainage, sanitation and waste clearance. At the District Council meetings he provided detailed and regular health reports. At the schools he cast an eye over all health issues, taking charge in the event of epidemics. Of course, all of this was severely challenging in the days of the horse and cart. Accidents and sicknesses could strike at any corner of his practice, and he would be expected to attend. No allowances could or would be made. This appointment also linked him closely to the Narberth Union, where the strict environment of the old workhouse added another dimension to his varied days.

The workhouse at Narberth dated back to the late 1830s, when the premises were purposely built at a site called Narberth Mountain, but today known as Allensbank. It is there that many of the poor people were housed in long narrow parallel stone buildings, which gave rise to natural court-yards. In Dr Creswick Williams' days, and much later still, the establishment was comprised of wards; kitchens and washing rooms; day rooms and dining areas; school teacher classes, and the master's living quarters.[17] Like other workhouses of its kind across the country, its overall functions were administered by a Board of Guardians. In the boardroom of its northern block, every fortnight, meetings would be held when the Master of the Union reported to the Board of Guardians on a range of issues – one of which now directly involved Dr Creswick Williams.[18]

The meetings were well attended and many subjects were discussed: inmates recently admitted; paupers, vagrants and tramps relieved; the monetary cost of providing relief; the financial contributions owed by the parishes, and any issues raised by the matron. There were reports on religious services held, visits from the general public, and gifts donated: often tobacco for the men, fruit and books for women and children. But one of the most important functions of the Board of Guardians was to appoint and oversee the medical officers

17 Narberth Workhouse and Poor Law Union Website – as at March 1st 2011.
18 *The Welshman*, 4 December, 1903, Carmarthenshire Archives Service.

of the designated districts, who would attend to the inmates – and it was at the boardroom of this historic setting that Dr Creswick Williams was offered the job that January day.[19]

Quickly attending to his duties, with no time to waste, Dr Creswick Williams rallied to every medical cause, sickness, accident and complaint. He gave his time, did his work, and moved on. There was no stopping now, medicine was in perpetual motion; it never left his thoughts. Others, too, were exploring this great subject day and night. Doctors were, after all, practitioners – learning, studying and taking medical advancements into new territories. Dr Creswick Williams had a fascination for herbal remedies. Botany was a favourite subject of his and a variety of different plant species were within his reach at the lowland, upland and sea locations. Medicinal herbs were important: foxgloves were now used for heart conditions; coltsfoot for chests, and coughs, and most doctors had their own favourites for different circumstances.

With the medical authorities encouraging doctors to share their discoveries with others, a comprehensive letter from Dr Creswick Williams appeared in *The Lancet* on March 3rd 1894, detailing the treatment he provided for a young patient. Other doctors did likewise, because improved health was everyone's genuine goal. The local and national papers played their part with regular doctors' columns. Also, advertisements for mixtures, ointments, and tablets were regularly featured – for ailments ranging from coughs and colds, to back and kidney problems, and more. Beecham's Pills was a favourite and they were well marketed, too. Besides appearing in the newspapers, advertisements cropped up where least expected, often on the side of wooden bathing carts that were rolled into the sea: 'Beecham's Pills Save the Doctor's Bills.'

---

19 *The Welshman,* 23 January, 1892, Carmarthenshire Archives Service.

As regards home visits, the trains, especially the Cardi Bach, helped enormously – a vital link to villages north of Whitland – while the horse and carts did the rest. Horses were well looked after and were the source of major employment. Besides farriers and blacksmiths, wheelwrights and saddlers, there were tanners, coachmen, stable hands and servants, whilst regular stopping places for the horses were situated at the roadsides. The Traveller's Rest Inn, between Whitland and Llanboidy, was one of these convenient halts.

Dr Creswick Williams built up a trusted relationship with the local Board School at Whitland – as well as with other schools all around the district, whose teachers called him for advice. The Log Book extract below is typical of so many provided by him at times of various epidemics:

> In consequence of the prevalence of Scarlet Fever amongst several of the children of Whitland, I consider it advisable to recommend the closure of The Board School for a period of at least three weeks.
>
> J. T. Creswick Williams
> Medical Officer for Health, October 19th 1899

Understandably, Dr Creswick Williams became a hugely respected public figure in Whitland, constantly in demand, and also supporting community events. But, if ever he wanted a peaceful moment, he had only to walk down to the meadow of his home, Prospect House, and sit on the river bank, listening to the running water. His residence was conveniently placed in the town – just like the fulcrum of his cartwheel – for the station, shops and stores. More importantly it was central for his practice.

Before its surgery days, Prospect House had been occupied, around 1891, by a corn merchant, his wife, eight children, and a servant.[20] Now it catered for patients, and countless people calling with messages for the doctor. From the front of the building, Dr Creswick Williams could look out of his consulting room window and see the school assembly taking place on the front yard beyond the railings. At different times of the day, he also heard the bell sounding high up in its beautiful bell tower. It had a distinct light tone, and when it rang to signal the resumption of classes, all the excitement and cheering that echoed around the playground fell silent.

20 British Census of 1891, Carmarthenshire Archives Service.

Marriage to Emily –
and a Mountain of Work

I N SEPTEMBER 1900, Dr Creswick Williams, taking a brief break from his duties, joined members and friends of St Mary's Church on a train outing to Rosebush in Pembrokeshire. After arriving, and having been 'fortified by buns and milk for the arduous climb,' they walked towards the top of the Preseli Mountains, where everyone spent a pleasant afternoon. Later, after supervising the children with organised races, for which the doctor was publicly thanked, they returned to the Preseli Hotel for tea.[21]

It was exactly a year later, in September 1901, that Dr Creswick Williams returned to this same peaceful part of the world to marry Miss Emily Margaret Carver, who, at the time, was a spinster of Mathry parish. This brought great excitement in the village of Mathry, and the town of Whitland – making headlines the next day, September 18th 1901, in the *County Echo, Fishguard and North Pembrokeshire, Advertiser:*

FASHIONABLE WEDDING AT MATHRY

At the Holy Martyr's Church, Mathry, on Tuesday last an interesting wedding took place between Dr J. T. Creswick Williams, Whitland, second son of the late Mr John Williams, formerly of Dolgellau, and Miss Emily Carver, daughter of Mr H. G. Carver JP, Blaencorse, St Clears, Carmarthenshire.

---

21 *The Welshman*, 21 September, 1900, Carmarthenshire Archives Service.

The ceremony was performed by the Reverend David Griffiths, vicar (brother-in-law of the bride).

The article mentioned that there had been a large and colourful congregation in attendance and the best man was Mr D. R. H. Thomas, a solicitor in Whitland. Miss Thomas, of Parke, (cousin) and Miss Griffiths (niece) were the two bridesmaids. After a reception at the Vicarage, the bride and bridegroom left this happy village scene for a traditional British beach honeymoon in Devon and Cornwall.

In *The Welshman* of September 27th 1901, there was a report on the newly-wed couple as they went on their way:

> On passing through Whitland, they were met at the railway station, and were given a grand reception by the leading inhabitants of the town. But that, and the booming of guns, was but a slight indication of the reception that will be in store for them when they return home on October 3rd – when the pupils of the Board and Intermediate schools, will be invited to tea, and a grand display of fireworks and rejoicings will add to the festivities of the day.

When the day arrived, *The Welshman,* of October 10th, stated that 'triumphant arches' had been put in place along the road leading to their surgery home, Prospect House. Tea was served across the road at the Board School, before the children 'marched in procession' to the station where a large crowd had gathered to await their arrival. There they entered a carriage – but it was not horse-drawn. No, this time they were given the silver-service of all honours; they were pulled by the people themselves:

> The vehicle was drawn through the streets of the town by many willing hands, and complimentary speeches were made at various points.

There would have been a warm welcome at the surgery home, too. Dr Creswick Williams had his own small team in place by now, including Martha Jane Owen, cook and domestic worker, and her sister, Margaret Mary Owen, housemaid. They dutifully attended to the housework and cleaning, while a general male servant was employed to look after the doctor's horse and stables. Martha Jane Owen – but known as Jane – is the grandmother of Yvonne Evans and June George, two sisters whose family originate from Whitland. Yvonne, who today lives at Efailwen, has a story to tell:

> My grandmother was very proud of her time with Dr Williams. Whilst working at his surgery home, she went to evening classes to learn cookery at the new County Intermediate School in North Road. She went there to improve the menu for the doctor. My grandmother was not used to presenting a doctor with fancy food; she only knew about ordinary farming food. I still have the book with all the old-fashioned recipes.
>
> Both my grandmother and her sister were from Market Street, where their parents lived at the time, but they never seemed to go home. They spent all their time at the surgery, sleeping there, too. I imagine they were kept busy answering the door to callers. No doubt, people were regularly leaving messages for the doctor to call.
>
> In 1904, my grandmother got married and she was given two large oil paintings by Dr and Mrs Williams. She told me that a visitor had painted these for the doctor, someone who was a guest at the house.
>
> Following her marriage she left the surgery to support her husband. This created a vacancy for another single girl, as was the custom of the day. No doubt, she was another Welsh speaker, because all Dr Williams' staff spoke Welsh.

Of course, his Welsh would have been strong, too, coming from north Wales.

My grandmother also referred to the old vicarage in Spring Gardens. This is where she worked before moving down the road to the surgery.

Today, Yvonne and her sister, June, are the proud owners of the oil paintings. One is a scene from the bottom of the Dolycwrt meadow near the river at sunrise, and the other is a scene from Esther's Ddôl, Afon Gronw – meaning Esther's house, *The Meadow*, on the River Gronw. This appears to be in Llanboidy, when, at the time of the painting, the river, seemingly, had burst its banks. Dr Creswick Williams was clearly fond of the river Gronw, which marked the eastern boundary of his garden. Indeed, this was evident from a statement made by Mr W. D. Davies many years later in 1968, in the fifth official programme of Whitland Week:

> When the South West Wales River Board carried out dredging operations to the River Gronw ten years ago, there disappeared from Parc Dr Owen a bathing pool which was regularly used by the late Dr Creswick Williams, who practised at Dolycwrt before Dr Owen.

If, upon getting married, Dr Creswick Williams' former housemaid needed a bank account, she would see that Lloyds Bank Limited had moved from its small sub-branch a few doors away to a prime location in the middle of St John Street.[22] There, it could compete with National Provincial Bank – situated at the time in King Edward Street – which had arrived two years earlier. Nearby, the building of the rather grand Public Hall, to be renamed Whitland Town Hall, King Edward Street, was also nearing completion that same

---

22 Lloyds Bank Group, Archives Department, London.

year, 1904. Indeed, the town was growing and, no doubt, Dr Creswick Williams' patients list was growing, too.

Whitland railway station was thriving now, bringing in greater volumes of passengers in the chocolate and cream-coloured carriages. Freight delivery never stopped: stone, slate, coal, timber and farm produce all arriving in heavy wagons, bearing the names of local traders painted on their sides. There was never a dull moment, people coming and going, tasks needing to be performed, lad porters running around trying to please everyone – while, outside, horse and carts pulled into and out of the Station Square all day long.

As part of their overall responsibilities, it was not unusual for country doctors, such as Dr Creswick Williams, to remove the occasional tooth during times of need. Now, however, Whitland's conscientious doctor would have taken delight in knowing that a dentist had arrived in town. With his multitude of tasks, Dr Creswick Williams needed every available assistance, and the arrival of Messrs Walker and Tew in St John Street, each Friday, between noon and 4pm, was seen by him as a positive and most welcome addition to the town's medical facilities.[23]

In his never-ending efforts to promote improvements in health and to support his profession, Dr Creswick Williams liked to help influence its direction, too. In the summer months of July 1904 he jumped aboard the Great Western Railway train bound for Llanelli, where he attended the annual meeting of the regional branch of the British Medical Association. It was held at Stepney Hotel, and *The Welshman* of July 15th recorded Dr Creswick Williams' proposal:

---

23 *The Welshman*, 23 October, 1903, Carmarthenshire Archives Service.

It was resolved on the proposition of Dr Creswick Williams, seconded by Dr Hopkin, that in the opinion of this meeting the time has arrived when the Association should undertake the defence of its members.

The paper also captured another important motion from the same meeting, which would later impact greatly on future medical students across the principality. It was decided that the local branch:

> heartily approved of the application to a supplemental charter to enable the University of Wales to grant degrees in medicine and surgery, and hereby records its opinion that under such a charter much benefit could accrue to the people of Wales.

Dr Creswick Williams returned home to a mountain of work. In addition to his growing private practice, his considerable duties as Medical Officer for Health were demanding more and more of his time. He was then giving his attention to St John Street, where he was troubled by piles of manure situated near the station. At a time when the roads were clearly being littered with the droppings of passing horses – acceptable then, and often collected by eager gardeners with a hand shovel and bucket – Dr Creswick Williams could not condone unnecessary health hazards such as he was now seeing. They could be the cause of all sorts of drainage and pollution problems which he had worked tirelessly to overcome, ever since he arrived in the town.

In fact, Dr Creswick Williams had previously aired his views on the subject – to the Rural Sanitary Authority of the Narberth Union – which appeared in the Medical Officer's Report Book,[24] as detailed below:

---

24 Carmarthenshire Archives Service.

Gentlemen,

With reference to the circular from the Local Government Board upon the probable occurrence of Cholera, I beg to report that so far as the 'No. 4 District' of the Narberth Union is concerned, the most necessary measures to be taken are:

1) Examination of the source of water supply, especially with regard to the danger of contamination of wells by sewage from the rivers.

2) The removal, under the Inspector of Nuisance, of all sewage heaps, and the disinfection of the places in which they stand, and the issue of caution upon the necessity of cleanliness and the liberal use of white wash upon pig sties and out buildings and stables.

3) The provision of an ample supply of ordinary disinfectants, especially chlorides of lime and carbolic acid and green copper, as for gratuitous distribution. The issue of white lime may also be advisable.

I desire to emphasise at this juncture, the urgent need of dealing with the filthy condition of the lane at the back of St John Street, Whitland. At present, refuse of all kinds especially manure from stables and pig sties is allowed to remain on the road and no drainage is provided.

A surer means of propagating disease cannot be imagined. I trust the authority will, at once, take steps to place the lane in a clean and healthy condition.

Dr Creswick Williams made one further point of considerable importance:

I would recommend that at some convenient spot in the Union, a building be provided which may, upon an emergency, be used as a hospital for infectious disease.

Anxious to see progress made, Dr Creswick Williams then wrote a separate letter to the Narberth Rural Sanitary Authority:

Gentlemen

Whitland Water Supply

There are two sources in the parish of Cyffig from which water could be obtained. One is close to a cottage called Cwm Colley, and the other from Cefn Coch.[25] I am informed that there is also water to be had on Mr Yelverton's property close to Whitland.

I should be pleased to meet any members of the Rural Sanitary Authority, and their Inspector, and accompany them so as to examine the different sources.

J.T.C.W.

Whitland's position, low down in the valley, was a major drainage concern. In 1898, the year that Dr Creswick Williams purchased Prospect House, he had been asked to produce a special report, which was again recorded in the Medical Officer's Report Book. He took into consideration the culverts in Cross Street; the needs for paving in Market Street; replacing the drains to the east of Pwllywhead Road; introducing a possible new scheme in North Road, and the general lack of 'fall' that affected most of the town streets, because the water simply could not run away.

No doubt, the problems that Dr Creswick Williams faced then were similar to many of his professional colleagues in rural areas – getting suggestions implemented. This was a slow process, requiring money and means. When making his annual report at the Parke Temperance Hotel (later named the Grosvenor Hotel), as reported in *The Welshman* of April

---

25 This is today better known as Cavan Coch.

14th 1899, it appears as though his patience had run-out concerning issues requiring attention in Park Street:

> Dr Williams said that in each annual report he had drawn their attention to that street. They must remember that the only public pump they had in Whitland was there, and, within a few hundred yards of it, all the filth and accumulation of ashes in the place were deposited there. It was really a disgrace that the street was kept in that way. It was a source of danger to the children in that neighbourhood, because when they went to school they were up to their ankles in water and remained in their wet boots all day long.

In his own words, Dr Creswick Williams could not be more succinct:

> I have wasted more ink and paper than would cover the road over, and nothing whatsoever has been done.

Not surprisingly, it was probably a relief for the hard working doctor to point his horse and cart in the direction of the open countryside to do some routine visits. There he could enjoy the hills and dales, as he made his way around the quiet country lanes. He would notice the original thatched cottages, knowing that, now in 1905, all new building work was being designed to very different plans.

It was around this time that Dr Creswick Williams was asked to attend a consultation with Dr Rowley Thomas in his native Henllan Amgoed. No doubt, he would find this a refreshing experience, because Dr Thomas was so likable and humorous. Then, a little while later, he repaid the compliment, asking Dr Thomas to assist him when a boy fell off his horse at Velfrey Road, in Whitland.[26] There was no end to the work of Whitland's popular doctor; there was no end to the variety of his duties, either.

---

26 *The Welshman,* 21 July, 1905, Carmarthenshire Archives Service.

A Nurse arrives
as Dr Creswick Williams departs

URING HIS TIME in Whitland, Dr Creswick Williams had enjoyed the friendship of another country doctor, who practiced medicine from his surgery home, five miles away. This was Dr Vaughan Daniel Williams Bowen-Jones, of Glan-yr-Afon, Lower Village, Llanboidy. These two gentlemen, highly placed in their respected communities, shared confidences and opinions about their patients. From Glan-yr-Afon they would occasionally wander down the peaceful country lanes, discussing the latest news and events. Indeed, with the years passing by so quickly, there would be a lot to discuss.

By now, Robert Koch's earlier work on the dreaded tuberculosis had led to further findings, aspirin was readily for sale, and modern practices in surgery were making progress. The passing of Dr Barnardo, who generously left his homes for orphans, and the wonderful Florence Nightingale, would sadden the two doctors – whilst away from medicine, there were more exciting stories: Henry Ford's new cars; Rolls Royce motor vehicles; Marconi's wireless signals; Lusitania's record Atlantic crossing, and Louis Bleriot's flight across the English Channel. Suddenly barriers were being pushed back, as the world opened up for all to see. Transportation and communication were advancing in leaps and bounds and the two doctors knew that this would have a great impact upon medical advancements too.

Dr Bowen-Jones' daughter, Mrs Caroline Rees-Davies, is alive today, aged 98. She can remember the old days when she had a rather privileged upbringing in Llanboidy's quiet country setting, where she attended the local school. Caroline can remember her father treating patients in the back room, and meticulously mixing medicines in his own dispensary:

> I certainly knew of Dr Creswick Williams. When I was a young girl his widow, Emily, used to call at Glan-yr-Afon with her mother. They would often stay with us. We were all good friends.
>
> Both my father and Dr Creswick Williams were proud of their profession and their surgeries. I can remember patients entering Glan-yr-Afon through the back door, sometimes calling because of tooth ache. Visiting a doctor's house was a big thing for patients in those days. People were often in awe of the doctors, because they were so important. They tried their hardest for everyone. There were far less distractions then, of course, and medicine filled their lives.
>
> In those days we used to have hanging oil lamps in Glan-yr-Afon. Being a doctor's daughter, many people expected me to go away to school, but my father was keen that I joined the children in Llanboidy.
>
> One of my earliest memories as a little girl concerned the Titanic. I remember it being in my mind because it sunk in April and I was born in November. When I was growing up, it was talked about for years. It was such a disaster that, almost every day, something was said about it. My father had *The Sphere* publication, and there was terrific coverage in those great big pages.

In October 1912, Dr Creswick Williams was called to Whitland's Railway Tavern (today's Taf Hotel), because a drover of no permanent address had fallen outside the pub. The local police constable saw this happen and duly summoned help. Dr Creswick Williams put the limb back in place, before referring this patient to his former employers at Carmarthen;[27]

> Mr Griffiths, Railway Tavern, with his customary good disposition, allowed the patient to stay in his house during the night, supplying him with all the necessary comforts, and attended to him assiduously . . . On the following day he was taken by train to the Carmarthen Infirmary, where, undoubtedly, he will receive the very best possible attention, coupled with scientific skill.

The next month, Whitland welcomed a nurse to the town. It was Nurse Edwards from Morriston, and a grand reception and tea was arranged at the Town Hall to mark this important occasion. Dr Creswick Williams was there helping the young nurse to feel at home and to make acquaintances. Dr Rowley Thomas, the chairman, expressed his delight at her arrival, adding just a few words of his customary, and well received, humour:

> He had known Miss Edwards since she was a little child when he had much affection for her, and although she was now a full grown lady, he thought he still loved her. A capable nurse was a good help to the medical man, especially one possessing the qualifications of Nurse Edwards.[28]

In early March 1913, St David's Day was celebrated in truly patriotic style in Whitland with an evening dinner at the Parke Temperance Hotel. Both ladies and gentlemen were in attendance, and there were performing artists and speakers between the serving of food. Dr Rowley Thomas was one,

---

27 *The Welshman*, 25 October, 1912, Carmarthenshire Archives Service.
28 *The Welshman*, 1 November, 1912, Carmarthenshire Archives Service.

interesting and humorous as always, describing his early days in London. Coordinating the event as chairman was Dr Creswick Williams, who welcomed the Bard of Brynach as the main guest. There were many toasts, including one to the Army, Navy and Auxiliary Forces. After seeking permission from the ladies for the gentlemen to smoke, the King and Royal Family were toasted by Dr Creswick Williams . . .

> . . . who said that he was pleased to observe that the King was following in the footsteps of his father. He added that our present ruler was a good one and did not interfere with political matters as his cousin across the channel did in such a perfunctory manner. Our King was not a warrior politician, actor or preacher, but a sound English gentleman, who was respected throughout the world.

Dr Creswick Williams was referring to Kaiser Wilhelm II of Germany; clearly, the events of an impending war were on everybody's minds. But the doctor also had a family worry to contend with at the time, because his wife's mother was unwell. Since being taken into their home, this popular lady's health had weakened, and she later died.[29] The funeral cortège left the surgery-house, passing the little school before heading out of Whitland into the narrow country lanes for Blaencorse, the lady's former residence. Mrs Carver was buried at the nearby village church in Llangynin, with gently rolling countryside all around. There are three small steps near the entrance where, probably, horses were mounted during these times. They may have reminded the doctor of his own intentions to step down from work – because he was already planning his retirement. At this stage, it was a well-guarded secret, but soon it was to be revealed to all.

---

29 *The Welshman*, 4 July, 1913, Carmarthenshire Archives Service.

The news came as a big shock around the town, and the district, and the board room of the Narberth Union; and the committee room of the Parke Temperance Hotel, where the district councillors met. Dr Creswick Williams was not only retiring, but he was retiring because of ill health. The announcement was hardly easy for the great physician, yet he handled it with his usual dignity. Heading into his 57th year, sadly, retirement was upon him. He was too proud and professional to cause alarm in the community by prematurely revealing his intentions to leave. Having made up his mind, he planned his every move before making this decision known, including choosing a successor. Then his official announcement was delivered by letter at the local council meeting, as reported in *The Welshman,* of September 12th 1913:

MEDICAL OFFICER RESIGNS

A letter was received from Dr Creswick Williams stating that, owing to the state of his health, he was obliged to relinquish his practice. He thanked them for the kindness they had shown him, and tendered his resignation as Medical Officer. His general practice would be taken over by Dr W. D. Owen, and he hoped that the Council would appoint Dr Owen as the Medical Officer for Health.

Sitting behind his large oak desk in the front consulting room, with a doctor's couch nearby, Dr Creswick Williams would feel great sadness leaving so much behind. In this, the twilight hour of his medical day, the memories of Plymouth Ironworks, Aberaman, the County Infirmary, and all the great medical establishments in London, would enter into his thoughts. But it was here in Whitland that he enjoyed his greatest days: living and breathing medicine, in his own surgery-home. He would be leaving behind a few treasured books from his personal library: one being *Secret Remedies*, 1909 (British Medical Association, London), where at the top of page 52, under a paragraph entitled 'Hamm's Rheumatic, Gout, and Sciatica Cure,' he had boldly written in clear black ink 'J.T.C.W. 18 Oct 09.' Indeed, Dr Creswick Williams' contributions to local medicine had been considerable, and his legacies would be great.

Whitland now had a dedicated surgery, whose doors were open to the public, and where patients could call to see the doctor, or to request a visit. Although only fifteen years into its tenure as a surgery, it would one day live on to complete a remarkable full and rounded century. But it was no longer Prospect House. Dr Creswick Williams had seen to this. Its new name was Dolycwrt; it was married to 'Medicine' now, and Dolycwrt was its medical name. Translated into English, it describes a meadow where there is a courtyard. This is a suitable description, because there is a natural courtyard at the back of the house between the old stable and the castellated perimeter walls.

Throughout Whitland and its outlying community, Dr Creswick Williams' departure would be sorely felt. With his quiet, easy, and assured manner he brought all that was great concerning patient care to this wide country practice. It is true that his legacy went further, because he had given a highly respected local boy the chance of taking over his private practice, whilst also recommending his appointment as Medical Officer for Health. After attending to all resignations and formalities, Dr John Thomas Creswick Williams quietly left the scene in September 1913. He and his wife, Emily – for medicinal purposes – were leaving in search of the fresh sea air and retirement at Borth, in Cardiganshire.

Reaching out for a Special Medical Baton

A T THE HOUSE SURGEON'S residence in the old King Edward VII Hospital, Cardiff, in the late summer of 1913, a young and recently qualified doctor was planning to return to his native homeland in west Wales. Dr William David Owen MB, BS (Lond), MRCS (Eng), LRCP (Lond., St. Barts) was enjoying his role in the Eye, Ear, Nose and Throat Department of this famous hospital,[30] a stunning landmark alongside the road leading to Newport from the city centre. This was another medical building of immense character and importance, with a most appealing stone frontage, and it was to be affectionately known, in later years, as Cardiff Royal Infirmary.

Dr Owen was a fashionable young man and Cardiff had so much to offer him. James Howell's store, the recognised family outfitters, had already become established and was soon to expand from the Hayes into St Mary's Street[31] and the sport he loved most, cricket, had welcomed the Minor Counties matches to the Cardiff Arms Park earlier that summer. If he had stayed in Cardiff, and his heavy work load had permitted, there would be interesting days ahead. However, he knew about the Dolycwrt practice, and the special homecoming that awaited him. This would be a thoroughly challenging medical appointment, one that would fill his life with responsibility, immense duty and happiness for years to come.

---

30 *The Medical Directory,* The Royal College of Physicians Information Centre.
31 Howells Department Store, Wikipedia web site, as at March 1st 2011.

Since growing up as a young boy in Whitland, Dr Owen had known Dr Creswick Williams, just as everybody else in the town had known him. He remembered seeing him call at the local schools, attending to his work and politely moving on. More importantly, the old doctor was a family friend, he knew his father well, having attended many of the social events together for two decades. It would be hard for him to imagine Whitland without Dr Creswick Williams; equally it was difficult to comprehend filling the great doctor's shoes at such a young age. Now 25, but highly qualified and recommended, Dr Owen could not let this opportunity pass him by. Indeed, he would not think twice. He belonged to Whitland, where his roots were firmly planted; soon he would be the new family doctor in town.

The young William David Owen was the son of a well-known chemist, Mr Philip Owen, and his wife, Mary.[32] They ran their successful business from the Medical Hall premises, St John Street, in the heart of the town. His father had a strong agricultural background, being raised just a few miles into the outlying countryside, and he involved himself selflessly in many of the town activities. He worked tirelessly at Medical Hall, ensuring that all manner of mixtures, minerals, malts, syrups, balsams, liniments, salts and soaps were in stock and neatly arranged around the store. The beautiful glass bottles – most with cork or glass tops and narrow necks – filled the shelves in a sequence of varying colours, shapes and sizes. Mr Owen took delight in helping the local people when they needed a mixture and, no doubt, this had a bearing on his son's career choice, at an early age.

After moving through the classes and completing his schooling, the serious work began in the Smithfield area of

32 Birth Certificate, Registrar of Births, Marriages and Deaths, Carmarthen.

London, at the historic St. Bartholomew's Hospital. Also known as 'St. Barts' it is one of England's oldest hospitals dating back nearly 900 years.[33] Indeed, in its colourful past, it witnessed Henry VIII's personal contributions, and later the heavy destruction of the Great Fire of London, in 1666. Surviving the rigours of medical school took great discipline and dedication, but William David Owen, striving to keep on track, would not fail to be inspired by the professional people presiding over his studies, especially the upstanding senior surgeons, whom he hurriedly followed around the wards. Lectures and patient care were unrelenting, but, at least at St Barts, he could escape to enjoy the attractions of London's city centre.

It would not be difficult for William David Owen to travel to most of London's famous sights including Westminster, where in 1911, the latter years of the young medic's studies, one of Wales' most famous political figures, David Lloyd George, was putting forward a revolutionary National Insurance Bill.[34] The proposed system – soon to help the lower paid workers in times of sickness and unemployment – would also herald the beginning of the comprehensive National Insurance System of later years. Medicine had never been more interesting. It was moving at a faster pace now, but the young student from Whitland was covering his ground.

As with any relay race, the change-over of batons is an important stage and not to be underestimated. One person slows down so that another can safely take possession: drop it, and there is a bad start. There were no hiccups here. The hand-over was as perfect as it was unique. Dr Owen's father had been Whitland's chemist long before Dr Creswick Williams

33 St. Bartholomew's Hospital website and Wikipedia as at March 1st 2011.
34 1911 National Insurance Act, website both as at March 1st 2011.

arrived in the town some twenty years earlier. Since then, they had both shared a love of the small town, and had given it their heart and soul. They were together at the Town Hall welcoming Nurse Edwards to Whitland not many months ago, and their homes, Medical Hall and Dolycwrt, were separated by just a short stretch of Market Street. Doubtless, they supported each other in their respective professions, too, and it would be a colossal coincidence if both had not seen this day coming and prepared for it. This extra pair of hands ensured that no baton was dropped.

There were formalities to complete because Dr Owen was buying a private practice. This had to be paid for; the premises had to be considered, and the patients had to be discussed. Together the two doctors would have visited the gentry, the ministers, and the business proprietors of the town, as well as the patients in greatest need. No doubt, they would have found time for conversations too. Away from the concerns of an undeniable arms race in Europe, people shared an immense interest in transport's great march forward. Over the previous ten years, the motor car industry had been a huge success. Dr Owen, a modern young man, would benefit greatly from these luxuries of the day – just like his predecessor may have done in more recent years. And, no doubt they both would have known that the popular new Morris Oxford had left its factory site at Cowley earlier that year.

Dr Owen – Manning the Medical Fort

Dr Owen did not waste a moment settling into his new role, while making Dolycwrt a permanent home for him and his wife. He took delight in helping people and acknowledged the privileges afforded by his profession. There were immense pleasures in healing. It was a special feeling seeing patients recover in front of his eyes. It brought humility and deep inner contentment, and this was enough to keep him going when sadness struck, and patients unavoidably passed away.

Every time he entered or left Dolycwrt, he would see the little school across the road. He became a regular and popular visitor at the premises, and each time he made an official visit, it was recorded in the school log book. There were fewer school holidays in those days, and, that summer, there was an amusing entry concerning the children. They were known to be absent during such times as harvesting and blackberry-picking, but this time they had another excuse:

> When the school bell rang, there were only 32 pupils in their places. The remainder did not turn up until 9.30. They had left the premises to see a wedding at Nazareth Baptist Chapel, and were under the impression that they could be excused, because the Infants Department staff and members were present.

For many years the Friday market, and the less frequent Tuesday livestock mart, had brought people to the bottom of Park Street. Since his return to the town, Dr Owen had noticed a little more activity at this same site than in previous years. This was because the small dairy enterprise, started two years earlier from modest beginnings in a galvanised shed, was taking off. This was a business destined for greater things, soon to rise above established small dairies, such as Cox's Milk Factory, whose outlets provided work around the locality. Indeed, one day it would scale the heights of greatness – and be recognised far and wide as Whitland Creamery – but, for now, it was simply known as Merlin's Dairies.[35]

The outcome of Dr Owen's application for the Medical Officer for Health position had been confirmed to him and, likewise, a short public announcement followed in the *Pembroke County Guardian and Cardigan Reporter* on Friday September 19th 1913

MEDICAL OFFICER APPOINTED

There were two applications for the post of medical officer and public vaccinator for the Whitland district, rendered vacant by the resignation through ill health of Dr Creswick Williams. They were from Dr Roland L. Thomas and Dr W. D. Owen, both of Whitland.

The article concluded that Dr Owen had been appointed. This role now linked him to the Narberth Union, and the fuller duties carried out by his predecessor. It was an appointment that he, too, would honour for many years.

Like Dr Creswick Williams, Dr Owen found the considerable demands of this office extremely stretching. Housing was an on-going major concern and he would often be asked to report on damp or unhealthy conditions, leakages, defects, walls out of alignment, indeed anything that impacted upon

---

35 Tapes of Tom Evans, former Milk Factory employee. Provided by Keith Thomas, former Factory Manager.

healthy living conditions. One of the earlier entries in the Medical Officer's Record Book during Dr Owen's tenure concerned houses in Llanfallteg, where another drainage problem had reared its ugly head. This time, work was to be carried out near the Railway public house, known today as the Plash Inn.[36] The roads, too, were causing all sorts of problems, not helped by the heavy traction engines. They made conditions dangerous for pedestrians and motorists, while the growing number of cyclists were, perhaps, in greatest danger.

Dr Owen, keeping abreast of local and national news since the outbreak of the Great War, was hit by a deluge of changes. As men arrived at Dolycwrt for check-ups and official medicals, before leaving for training centres across the country, others were heading straight into battle, leaving behind sad and desperate loved-ones on the station platform. In the family homes, farms, and work places, women filled the shoes of the departed men. Others joined the brave Women's Auxiliary Army, while local members of the British Red Cross Society actively promoted all war efforts – raising money, finding accommodation for the wounded, and seeking volunteers to help in every way.

As the state of warfare quickly heightened, the country required more and more doctors and surgeons, who, attached to the Royal Army Medical Corps, were sent abroad. Nurses would likewise be posted overseas, and this meant that Dr Owen and his colleagues on the home front would be actively manning the medical forts with depleted work forces. Indeed, they would be soldiering on themselves, faced with a never-ending schedule of demands. Dr Rowley Thomas, who had

---

36 *A History of a West Wales Village: Llanfallteg,* Llanfallteg History Society, ISBN 978-0-9562134 -0-2

already come to Dr Owen's assistance when performing a local operation shortly after he arrived at Dolycwrt, was soon to go away. Attached to the Welsh Horse Regiment, he was posted to Norfolk, before landing in the thick of fierce action in the Dardanelles.

Dr Owen, like so many others, would miss Dr Thomas. He was a colossal character in the town. Shortly before he left, he had presented oranges to the school children for Christmas. Likewise, he had played a big part in the early war meeting held in Whitland at the outbreak of hostilities. That night he represented the medical profession. During an evening which saw the male voice party singing *Comrades in Arms* and *Crossing the Planes* – and when appeals were made to the people of Whitland to provide money and men – the visiting speaker reminded everyone about the gravity of the war situation, as detailed in *The Welshman*, of August 18th 1914:

> Mr Peel said that the job in front of us was to put down, once and for all, the aggressive militarism of Germany. Through no fault of our own we were engaged in a titanic struggle with an ever-increasing world power, endeavouring by every means to become eventual master of Europe.

Dr Rowley Thomas was not the only member of his family preparing for battle. At this same time *The Welshman* published a light-humoured account that referred to Dr Thomas' well-recognised shooting skills. It concerned his wife's son, Mr Garbutt Hutchinson, who was also preparing to be posted overseas:

> It need hardly be added that he is an excellent shot, a qualification that will doubtless serve him in good stead whenever he comes in contact with some of the Germans.

Besides attending to his own patients, Dr Owen was now expected to help at other nearby practices and hospitals. Venues such as hotels, halls and temporary extensions within hospital grounds were all catering for injured soldiers, as were the Board of Guardians at the local Workhouses. Understandably, there was a big emphasis on training nurses, and arranging first aid classes – and there were many of these. Dr Owen gave every help to the local nurses from the beginning. He understood how vital they were in supporting his role as family doctor. He encouraged the Nursing Association in the district to remain strong, and this depended upon the locals giving generously towards the nurses' salaries.

In raising money for the war, the churches, chapels, schools and other organisations all played their part, while supporting each other's efforts united the entire community. It was important that fund-raising was coordinated by a separate single organisation, and a dynamic local committee, called the Whitland Soldiers and Sailors Fund, assumed this function. Likewise, the Whitland War Savings Association regularly held meetings to promote and encourage savings, and Dr Owen was often involved chairing these proceedings.

Dr Owen also attended the regular recruitment events that were staged in the town and the district. The visiting recruitment officers depended upon the local doctors being present to examine the recruits before they went to war. According to a report in *The Welshman*, at a specially arranged evening in Whitland Town Hall in December 1915, Dr Owen was present, when:

> fifty men from various parishes presented themselves, but ten were rejected as medically unfit. The other forty were duly attested.

Now, approaching Christmas 1915, time had marched on, and Lieutenant Hutchinson of the Welsh Horse Regiment, was serving abroad. Corresponding with his mother, in Henllan Amgoed, he described his early war experiences, which appeared in *The Welshman* on November 12th 1915. He described his safe landing overseas, when the soldiers, being so exhausted, just lay down and slept. He wrote about the Turkish trenches being nearby and the dysentery that they had overcome. Being on an isolated hillside location, he missed the simple things in life, like going to a shop. As a group of soldiers, excellent camaraderie prevailed among the men, who gathered to share a joke in the evening. In this brave and cheerful message, he hinted for more letters and a drop of whiskey, too. Then he commented on the enemy: describing the state of confusion that prevailed on the front lines, during this stubborn, senseless war:

> They seem very anxious to stop fighting, and most of them don't know what the row is about. It is just the German officers who keep things going.

Dr Owen, reading this at home in Dolycwrt, would clearly be moved by the hopelessness of these hostilities. Ever since Germany had invaded neutral Belgium, Britain, like its Commonwealth countries, had been locked in combat. The list of personnel heading into battle was colossal, and the number of casualties was immense. And it was hardly surprising that the effects of these distant upheavals were working their way back home, where Dr Owen would also be involved.

A Time of Sadness for Dr Owen

B ESIDES VISITING wounded soldiers during their convalescence, Dr Owen's wartime caring involved spending
considerable time with families who were suffering the
traumas of having relatives injured, or missing, in the fields of
battle. Every day, news filtered through of more casualties, as
anxious families awaited the morning post and newspapers
with a mixture of fearful emotions. Truly, this was a time of
immitigable sadness: a time when so many, so often, would
turn to the reverence of local churches and chapels for quiet
reflection and prayers, or to the consoling words of their
minister or doctor for encouragement. Everywhere, everyone
had to dig deep to find spirit and fight to hold on. Although
few people realised, this included Dr Owen as well. In the
midst of this great sadness, more bad news was making its
way into his surgery-home – firstly from the peaceful village
of Borth.

Dr Owen was aware that since Dr Creswick Williams'
retirement in the autumn of 1913, he and his wife, Emily, had
settled into Bay Ridge Villa,[37] a fine residence in Cliff Terrace,
which looked across the long beach towards Aberdyfi, a
few miles away. The doctor and his wife both thoroughly
enjoyed the healthy air, clear blue sea, miles of sand, and the
nearby dunes at Ynys-las. The fascinating and varied wildlife
of the Dyfi Estuary absorbed Dr Creswick Williams, the
botanist; and, likewise, Borth, with its cold stormy winters,

---

37 Death Certificate, Registry of Births, Marriages and Deaths.

had an interesting seafaring history. Dr Creswick Williams had known about the shipwrecks and the sunken forest that emerged at low tide. He also realised how important the herring catch was to the village, bringing great activity, especially during the autumn surf, when women and children lit bonfires to direct the fleet safely home.[38]

In the warmer summer sunshine, Borth – a fashionable, small, seaside resort with its own boarding houses – would burst into colour. Visitors, dressing up in smart costumes and hats, arrived regularly on foot, bicycle, or aboard the steam train that pulled into its small, Victorian station. It was an idyllic location for the doctor and his wife, who were preparing to settle into the larger Cliff Haven residence, only a few doors away. Sadly, however, their time together had come to an end. In a small extract from the full obituary appearing in the *Cambrian News and Welsh Farmers Gazette* on Friday June 2nd 1916, are the following tributary words:

DEATH OF DR CRESWICK WILLIAMS

He took a keen interest in Ambulance, Red Cross, First Aid and Nursing classes. His valuable services were recently recognised by the members making him a presentation. Dr Creswick Williams was highly respected at his adopted home and will be greatly missed by Borth people of all classes. For some years the deceased carried on a successful practice at Whitland, but owing to failing health, he retired to Borth about three years ago. During the last winter, he held large and successful Ambulance classes. The great number of people who attended the funeral testified to his popularity, and the respect in which he was held . . .

---

38 *Borth, a Seaborn Village,* Terry Davies, Gwasg Carreg Gwalch, ISBN 0-86381-877-3

To the very end this wonderful man gave his service. No doubt, his work for the Red Cross Society was his own personal contribution to this awful war. From the beach at Borth, the beautiful St Matthew's Church can be seen sitting on a ridge of higher ground decorated by trees. There, at his burial, the minister of Mathry, Rev. Griffiths – who conducted his wedding to Emily, in happier days – was one of the ministers officiating. Dr Creswick Williams rests with the Cambrian Mountains in the distance and the sound of the sea just a short step away. And on his tomb, for all to see, are the words . . . 'Formerly in Practice at Whitland.'

Dr Owen would not have fully absorbed this crushing news when, less than two months later, lightning struck for the second time. Now, his father had died: his lifetime friend, companion, guide, advocate – everything. Dr Owen's mother had passed away some nine years earlier, which had strengthened the bond between Dr Owen, his sister, Mildred, and their father. In such a short space of time Dr Owen's father and Dr Creswick Williams – the two people who had made it possible for him to practise at Dolycwrt – had gone. Talk about the ending of a triple alliance; here was another. It was a personal tragedy in the life of a young doctor, who was already carrying on his shoulders the burden of a broken-hearted community.

Dr Owen's father had spent forty years in business in Whitland, where he was loved and respected as the chemist. He saw at first hand the pain and suffering of local people who would arrive at his counter to buy his mixtures and tonics. Of course, in those days the doctors prescribed the stronger, more potent medicines but, throughout the years, Mr Owen played a major back-up role for the doctors, too. Indeed, he would often be the first to know who was unwell. Dr Creswick Williams knew exactly what he was doing for the town and community when he handed over the Dolycwrt reins to Dr Owen.

In his spare time, Mr Owen, the chemist, gave unreservedly to the community. The County Intermediate School, where his son was educated, was close to his heart, and he was so proud to be chairman of the Board of Governors. He was also a senior deacon at Tabernacle Chapel, and treasurer of Whitland Agricultural Society. It is understandable that *The Welshman* provided an outstanding obituary on August 4th 1916, describing the sad funeral service and burial at Soar Chapel. Indeed, some of the beautiful words of the reporter would have further touched the people of the community:

> He possessed much of the innocent and unassuming traits of a child, but closer intimation and knowledge of him revealed the qualities essential to form a very powerful personality. He rarely aspired to posts of honour or public fame although he was offered many, and whatever work he undertook, it was accomplished with accuracy and precision.

By the time Dr Owen and his sister, Mildred, had arranged for a beautiful ornamental cask to adorn their parents' tomb – a symbol of the old delftware pots used by chemists in earlier days – there was more sad news. Dr Rowley Thomas had been seriously injured on the border of Turkey. He arrived back in Whitland aboard a train, where people were distressed to see him a seriously injured man.[39] He had suffered injuries to both his shoulder and hip, and undertook a slow and steady period of convalescence.

It was not raining now; it was pouring. This time sadness came from Llanfyrnach, still within the boundary of Dr

---

39 *The Welshman*, 4 February, 1916, Carmarthenshire Archives Service.

Owen's vast practice, where William Thomas had lived before losing his life fighting for the country.[40] No doubt, this gentleman had one day jumped aboard the local train just a short stroll away from his cottage, Gwernant, full of hope and promise, ready and willing to play his part in the war – but he was not to return. Dr Owen would never know that the baby son of William, and his wife, Martha, would one day become a highly successful surgeon, working overseas in a number of distant countries. And, on the way, he would spend time as a locum in Dolycwrt in the early 1940s.

40 Conversation with Creselda Davies, Clynderwen, a relative.

A Return to Peacetime Practice

THE NEWS OF Dr Rowley Thomas' recovery was uplifting for the whole community; it was like a ray of light. However, he did not return to local practice immediately, because he was soon on his way to Egypt, for more war service as a hospital surgeon.[41] There was no stopping Dr Thomas. He was setting a wonderful example, playing his part heroically, every step of the way. Indeed, so many people were, each offering different contributions – including Lena Guilbert Ford, whose medicinal tonic *Keep the Home Fires Burning,* seemed to have come straight from the dispensary. It had been a long and awful few years, but the end signalled relief, and peace and harmony, despite the considerable set-backs and grief that had to be overcome.

At this stage many soldiers and prisoners of war had not yet been released or discharged from duty abroad. They were all waiting patiently in distant parts for their great moment, malnourished, and only a shadow of their former selves. On account of this, the town's fund-raising and the war savings did not stop. In the early months of the New Year 1919, a Victory Ball was staged at Whitland Town Hall.[42] This set the trend for a hectic social calendar, as presentations and welcome-home parties became regular events. All military personnel, whatever their rank and file, were treated to the warmth of an official reception in their honour, and, on many

41 *The Welshman,* 3 September, 1916, Carmarthenshire Archives Service.
42 *The Welshman,* 31 January, 1919, Carmarthenshire Archives Service.

occasions, Dr Owen undertook the duties of toastmaster, or guest speaker.

One of these parties was held for Dr Rowley Thomas. *The Welshman* of February 15th 1918 tells the story of his return. Having earlier been treated to a special tea at the delightful little country school in Henllan Amgoed,[43] just a walk up the road from his farm residence, another reception awaited him at the Whitland Council School, where he was warmly welcomed by the Soldiers and Sailors Welfare Committee:

> Mr Rogers, West Regwm, said it was a great sacrifice for the doctor to enlist and leave all behind, especially the hounds and the foxes, as they knew what a great sports-man he was.
>
> Dr Thomas, in thanking them, said he had been with the Welsh Troops for over three years, and they were the bravest men in the world. He had been wounded himself and carried off the field. Of all four Fronts on which he had served, the Dardanelles was the worst, where such a high percentage of deaths were due to sicknesses.

It was around this time that another local war hero returned home, having been imprisoned in a German camp during the latter stages of the war. This was William John Llewellyn – known as Gwilym – whose son, John, is well known as former headmaster of both Henllan Amgoed, and Llanboidy schools. John explained that his father was returning to 14 Market Street, only a few doors away from Dolycwrt:

> When my father returned, he weighed just seven stones. He arrived back at a crowded Whitland Railway Station, and was carried shoulder high.

---

43 *The Welshman* – 24 January, 1919 and 15 February, 1918. Carmarthenshire Archives Service

During those days everybody was starving in Germany, and many of the Red Cross parcels didn't get through. As a result of this, my father suffered from a stomach complaint for many years.

Back in Whitland the local doctors were very keen. They spent as much time as possible with the soldiers, examining them physically, and helping them to rebuild their lives. I believe it was Dr Owen who attended to my father, referring him on to Tenby Cottage Hospital, where he had an operation . . . And it was a wonderful hospital, too. It was only small, but father said that it was really good there. And he was thrilled with the treatment he received.

Up the road in Llanboidy, Dr Bowen-Jones was also taking time to meet the returning soldiers of his country practice. His daughter, Caroline, explains:

My father took great interest in the men returning from the war. He made time to visit them, to help them settle back into the community. Many had experienced severe hardship and had been shocked. It was important that they were treated kindly . . . And he often joined the men in the local pub. He bought them drinks – this is what they liked – and the Maesgwynne Arms was the place to go at the time.

On Saturday July 19th 1919, Dr Owen would have been aware of the organised Peace Parade taking place near his front rooms at Dolycwrt, being Whitland's contribution to a national event. A banner carried the words 'Victory and Peace with Honour,' and a procession of children and adults made their way around the town, ending up at the Council School. It is there that everyone had tea on the lawn, followed by a sports event, before fire balloons brought the day to a colourful close.

Medicine was seeing the beginning of a new day. So much had been learnt from the fighting, and new avenues opened for research. Infections and diseases prevalent during the battles had to be explored; likewise, specialist hospitals offering orthopaedic and plastic surgery had emerged following the complicated nature of injuries. Dr Owen's knowledge of medical history had taught him that mankind, without medical knowledge and medicines had searched for whatever remedies could be found to assist the body's natural self-healing powers, even from prehistoric times. Faith and hope had played a huge part whilst the early 'discoveries and findings' continued into the 'medical research' of modern days. Indeed, here lies the golden thread of continuity, each succeeding generation having shone the light a little further.

Through professional bodies, such as the Royal Society of Medicine and the British Medical Association, communication channels to the doctors were now highly effective. For Dr Owen, journals such as the *Lancet* and the *Practitioner* arrived on the colourful floor tiling of Dolycwrt's front passageway, offering support and enlightening reading. With doctors sharing their own stories, this straight forward practice was advancing medicine to new heights. Indeed, when patients were still dying of serious uncontrollable epidemics, such as tuberculosis and influenza, few doctors could prise themselves away from their work. Healing patients brought a desire to do more, and success inspired success – especially at a time when they knew that they could make a difference.

Dr Owen typified this type of person, fully available to patients around the clock. It would not be unusual to see lights on at Dolycwrt at any hour, because confinements and emergencies, sickness and epidemics arrived in their own time, as well as accidents too – and there were plenty of these. During times when old-fashioned mechanical activity powered the railways, mills, quarries, farms and factories; and when most people rode a horse, or bicycle, or drove a cart; and when manual workers like blacksmiths and wheelwrights handled tools – it was inevitable that accidents could and would happen.

Dr Owen would now be encouraged by the help of local first-aid enthusiasts and nurses. Both had taken major leaps forward during the war years, and would provide invaluable future support for the busy doctor. However, little would escape Dr Owen's final touches and he was comforted in knowing that the County Infirmary in Carmarthen was just a short distance away in case of need.

Dr Owen lends a 'Sporting Hand' to a Busy Town

D R OWEN WAS determined that it was time for sport to return to the town. A rugby or football match at the end of the week would bring the townspeople together. It would enhance friendship, boost morale and lighten everybody's lives in this difficult post-war period. He was now playing a leading role in the formation of an athletic club in the town, and had chaired meetings held at the Yelverton Hotel. The local boys had responded well, too, raising a rugby team for a little excursion into Pembrokeshire, where they were to play Kilgetty, in the first round of the District Cup competition. This match, described in *The Welshman*, on March 26th 1920, was just one of a series of reports, detailing rugby's post-war return to Whitland. Below are extracts:

> When they last visited Kilgetty for a friendly game they sprang a surprise on the homesters, but they will probably find Kilgetty well prepared on Saturday. They leave Whitland by the 2.20 train and it is hoped that a large crowd of supporters will accompany them to cheer them on in the contest.
>
> September 1920, versus Tenby . . . 'When the forwards have more practice and experience, there is every reason to believe that the team will do well.'
>
> October 1920, versus Carmarthen Harlequins 2nd XV . . . 'The visitors were on the field ready to play, at the arranged

time, when people were still looking for men to play for Whitland.'

There were other matches too, including a contest which saw Whitland 'Old Crocks' beat the present players, highlighting the refreshing attitude to sport and rugby that prevailed at the time. And who could blame the rugby boys for being relaxed? They had jobs, they worked long hours, and the town was growing. Everyone could see this, because the shops were bursting with activity and new houses were being built. There were now enough financial transactions to keep four major Banks busy: Midland having become well-established and open for three days a week, covering Saturdays, market, and mart days, at premises in West Street.[44]

For years, the Friday Market, often referred to as the weekly Provisions Market, held at the bottom of Park Street, attracted the crowds, selling ducks, rabbits, geese, eggs, butter, as well as a variety of home-made items, such as thick rugs made in the countryside. Farmers and merchants travelled into town with their carts laden with produce; many more arrived by train. These were special occasions which nobody wanted to miss, as men, women and children walked and cycled, even in the wet and wintry weather to be involved. Meanwhile, for those who roamed around the countryside taking shelter in barns or hayricks, these gatherings offered warmth and activity which they, too, could enjoy.

Similarly, the Tuesday Livestock Marts, held at this same location – and the sheep sales staged at Stokesay's Field, near St Mary's Church – were bustling affairs, as animals descended upon the town from all directions. Often herded for miles along the country lanes, and coaxed into crowded pens amidst the cluttered confusion of the day, most would be heading to

44 HSBC Bank Archives Department.

the busier towns and cities at night. Meat dealers, butchers and farmers came from afar to bid for stock, whilst on the platform edge, stalls, enclosures and pens were prepared to direct the animals away. It was on days such as these that the adrenalin flowed under the auctioneer's hammer. And it was amongst the animals, farmers, shoppers – and the general merriment of the pubs – that the wheels of Whitland's rural economy turned round and round.

Witnessing such purposeful scenes in his native town pleased Dr Owen. His father had been a big lover of the country and, of course, a keen member of the Whitland Agricultural Show committee. The big crowds attending these events had brought bountiful trade to his father's shop, as well as a sense of real importance to the town. Of course, from Dolycwrt, Dr Owen would hear the sounds of the mart from the bottom of the street, and this often prompted him to take a stroll down the road, where he would soon be engulfed in all the activity.

Dr Owen knew that the town's progress impacted directly upon the surgery; a busy town would bring more inhabitants and more patients. For this reason he might have had mixed thoughts about two of the issues being discussed in the Whitland Parish Council meetings at this time. One concerned outside traders avoiding the payment of rates, while the other was the rather more serious health issue concerning animals wandering through the streets of Whitland on mart days. Both could have an impact on the surgery and its patients, too, as indicated in the minutes of the meeting held on July 5th 1922. Below is an extract:

The Parish Council are of the opinion that there should be a toll, and, if they are on private property, ask the District

Council to approach the owners so that payment be made, as in other towns.

Also, many farmers take their bulls to Whitland Mart without being led, which practice is dangerous to the public – and the Parish Council would be grateful if the District Council would see that this practice is done away with in the future.

For years the Great Western Railway had been a source of major employment, as well as providing players for the town football and rugby teams. Youngsters leaving school started as cleaners, with their work closely scrutinised before they rose through the ranks. Dr Owen was delighted to see Whitland's Station heading towards its glory days, complete with engine shed, turntable and two signal boxes, one east, one west. Now among the loads of produce arriving daily at the station, was milk delivered in heavy 17 gallon churns. These were filled in the early hours of the morning by farm servants and parlour maids milking by hand. And they were soon on the way to distant towns and cities but not until they had entered Whitland's growing factory, for its important seal of approval.

As summer approached in this same year, 1922, Dr Owen would have been amused to read a message from a local cricket enthusiast sent to *The Welshman,* and published on May 19th 1922. Village cricket then was such a socially accepted recreation, associated with park settings, green grass, smart white kit, hot summer weather, slow-paced bowling, and peacefulness – broken by the unmistakable sound of a leather ball hitting the white willow of a bat. Historically, matches had begun between rival parishes, and then large estates such as the old Maesgwynne Mansion Estate near Llanboidy, who had a team – and a traditional tea followed the play:

'May I encroach upon your space just to ask a little question of the Whitland Cricket Club committee? Where is the cricket club?' he had asked. 'Where has it gone to and when does it intend returning? After getting a suitable ground, the committee shows no desire to 'get a move on.' I have seen no one preparing a pitch, nor heard of any fixture arranged. Why, in the old days at Whitland, we had lost three or four matches by this time of year.'

The next week in the same paper, dated May 26th 1922, were the answers. Club members had held a general meeting and Mr Douglas Rees had been appointed to lead the Cricket XI, while Mr Roberts from Lloyds Bank was to be the vice captain. They had been asked to arrange a match. The captain's side was comprised of single men and Mr Roberts' side was to consist of married men. According to the paper, the outcome of this encounter was conclusive: 'the single men had by far the better of the argument.'

Dr Owen, taking a rest from medicine, had played. On this occasion, he failed to hit a run, but he had bowled well, with two of the opposition caught out from his deliveries.

Soon after the close of play, Dr Owen was back at work, spending time with his patients, a special quality that could not be bought or dispensed or prescribed. He was remembered for his gentle nature, natural kindness, support and encouragement; yet he could equally be assertive and forthright with his views.

He fought for the practice and his patients with determination, but always with the manners and eloquence of a gentleman. When he delivered his annual report as Medical Officer for Health in 1923, he had reminded everyone that there was no hospital in the area, no facilities for infectious diseases, and a shortage of midwives in the district. An extract from *The Welshman* dated September 14th 1923, reads as follows:

> I feel, and I am certain all members of the medical profession who have to attend cases in sparsely populated areas will agree, that the conditions that at present exist should not be tolerated any longer. I would suggest that the only way out of the difficulty is to select suitable women in the districts where they are needed, who are already resident in those districts, and to encourage them by granting subsidies to undergo a course of training at a suitable maternity school. It is only in this way that maternity cases in country districts can hope to receive the proper and adequate treatment which is meted out to them in the populous districts.

Only a few months later, Captain W. Griffiths, Canadian Emigration Agent for Wales, visited Whitland to give an address that was chaired by Dr Owen. At this time, un-employment across the country was seriously high. This was clearly a real social concern, causing unrest. Across Britain there had been disputes and industrial action, and national strikes would soon be taking place, which would also affect staff of Whitland Railway Station. Captain Griffiths had arrived to convey the simple message that jobs were both available and guaranteed in Canada.

Returning to his official health duties in the town, Dr Owen was now addressing a problem concerning the weekly sewage collection. It was 1924 and the horse and cart had for many years made nightly visits to the back lanes of Whit-land, taking away the contents of people's buckets into the countryside. From the Medical Officer's Record Book, it appeared that an additional lane was required. Whilst making these suggestions seemed straight forward, seeing the work completed was a different matter:

SPRING GARDENS BACK LANE

Suggested that a back lane (right of way) should be made, so as to enable the sewage cart to collect refuse from the rear of the houses. At present, the contents of the pails have to be deposited in the front – carried through the houses.

Certain owners object to paying a share of the money required for the purchase of land for such a lane.

When it came to the annual pleasure fair, however, nobody could disagree that this was a night of real entertainment in the town that everybody looked forward to. The Council School 'scholars,' as they were then called, were treated to a customary full-day's holiday, and crowds travelled many miles to enjoy the fairground attractions.

These were dark and often very wet nights, but they came action-packed with excitement, and young children often received a few pennies to spend from a good neighbour or friend – 'dyma ffeiryn bach i ti' ('here is a small present for you'), they would say. Above all else, these events were known as hiring fairs, because boy and maid servants were hired during these nights by the farmers. Howard Gibbon who can remember Dr Owen visiting his mother at the old farm cottage near his present home, explained:

When I was a child, Whitland Fair was always held on the last Friday in September, and it was called a 'hiring fair.' The 'hiring' took place anywhere in St John Street. But the 'pleasure fair' attractions were at Jimmy Lewis' field. He was a merchant selling eggs and poultry, and his shop is where the police station is today. The field was behind the shop on the site of the old dairies, factory – near to Dr Owen's Dolycwrt Surgery.

Boys and girls gathered in groups if they were looking to be employed. It would be more than a job then: it was an annual contract, and fair day marked the end of that contract. To secure the services of a good worker, farmers usually raised his or her salary. In this way, servants could secure the best wages for the coming year. They lived on the farms, and knew that they would not starve. The negotiations were finalised when the farmer gave the servant a piece of silver – usually half a crown – and this was to be given back if the promise was later broken.

During the fair nights, Dr Owen would have noticed small market stalls around the streets selling a variety of items. Traders and farmers would be selling their wares. At the time, boxing was a big interest with most boys of the town and organised fights would take place at the Fishers Arms, when the local boys would challenge visiting boxers.

With so much happening, fair nights could be busy nights for Dr Owen. Many people who came into Whitland with a few spare pennies in their pockets, spent this on booze. And some of them, inevitably, were not used to it. When they found themselves tumbling over and getting hurt, it was time to disturb Dr Owen – and I daresay this happened often.

In 1927, everyone in Whitland was proud to see work progressing with the Memorial Hall in Market Street, a fine spacious building replacing earlier temporary facilities, and giving honour to the fallen heroes of the Great War. It would be the centre of so many events, meetings and activities and it would be one of the town's finest assets, as it still is today. It was very appropriate that a splendid, although understandably stately, opening ceremony was held early in the next year, commemorated by an official programme, dated Wednesday, February 22nd 1928.

Dr Owen had been involved in this venture, but it was his fellow, Dr Rowley Thomas, who made the important address that day after John Hinds Esquire, Lord Lieutenant of Carmarthenshire, had declared the hall open. The programme described the sequence of events, which saw the relatives of the fallen entering the premises, followed by the ex-servicemen. After prayers, hymns, choral offerings by the children, the Last Post, a minute's silence, and the Reveille, the Memorial Hall Tablet was formerly accepted by the Trustees, before Dr Thomas made his speech.

That day, Dolycwrt, only a hundred yards away, would have seen crowds of people all intent upon sharing this precious and respectful moment in Whitland's history. Many people had lost their lives, and one of these was a nurse, Nurse Edith Cavell, who was shot by the Germans in Brussels in 1915. She is well remembered in the Memorial Hall as a 'True Daughter of the Empire'.

Having now set such high standards of excellence, the management committee, including Dr Owen, pressed ahead with equal efficiency in tendering the hall to various town organisations for its regular use. There was both a considerable response and demand, and, a few months later, a billiard room offered the town people, and its doctors, yet another sporting outlet, which they would enjoy for years to come.

The Joys of Country Practice

FOR SOME TIME, Dr Owen had been one of the comparatively few proud owners of a motor car. His earlier models were two-seaters, ideal to get around the quiet country lanes and long tracks leading to the farms. At this time, car manufacturing, of today's treasured vintage and antique models, was one of the country's proud and steady growth industries, and each model was beautifully designed. The Austin 7 Box Saloon was another favourite. Small, but sturdy, compact and cosy, it was cheeky and brimming with character.

Dr Owen would sit back and admire the scenery as he went on his calls. In those days there were no driving tests, or painted roads, or dual carriageways. Roads were usually rough gravel tracks, often with trench-like culverts to the side, which took the water away, like a little stream, in the heavy rain. The sturdy, cast iron, black and white road signs gave directions, while the immovable milestones sat close to the kerbs and hedges. Dr Owen often went along the Llanboidy road, up and down the open green hillsides, which rolled away into the distance. And, as he dropped down into Lower Village, the wheels would automatically halt alongside Glan-yr-Afon. The great link between the two medical residences had continued throughout Dr Owen's days, too, and Mrs Caroline Rees-Davies can remember the occasions well:

Dr Owen called at Glan-yr-Afon to sit down and have a cup of tea for two minutes; sometimes he would even take a sleep. Then he would get up suddenly and be on his way: 'I must go.' He was kind, generous, a friend to trust, compassionate. He listened to people and we looked forward to his visits.

In the late 1920s, Dr Owen was called to Tre Howell, Glandŵr, because a small child aged three had double-pneumonia. Although penicillin had now been discovered, it would be years later before it could be prescribed, so the tried and trusted remedies of old were put in place. In the bedroom of this small cottage, the child was wrapped in cotton wool, whilst a piping hot coal fire heated both a kettle and pan of water to steam the room. Assisting Dr Owen at this time was a gentleman named Dr Llewellyn, and one of these two physicians returned to the child twice daily, encouraging her mother to gather flowers from the hedgerow to stimulate the small patient.

This is Rhiannon Jones, today a proud great-grandmother aged 84, who is the niece of Mary Myfanwy Jones, known as Mannie, who used to help Dr Owen at Dolycwrt. Rhiannon, who has a tale to tell about Mannie – Mrs Francis after marriage – remembers Glandŵr as a thriving little village. It had its own carpenter, blacksmith, mason, and cobbler, and the mill was beyond the village school. Everyone wore clothes made by the local tailor, and the children went to school in clogs. Rhiannon, just like her school friends, would tug away at the metal supports underneath her footwear when they came loose. This gave her an excuse to go down to the cobbler, who worked alongside the station platform, to see the trains coming in:

My aunt Mannie was employed by Dr and Mrs Owen at Dolycwrt, where she lived and did general home help. She thought the world of them both. They were very kind and gave her a dinner set for her wedding in 1936. I remember Mannie telling me that, when Dr Owen died a year later, she continued to help Mrs Owen, and they became close friends. When Mannie later left her employment, Mrs Owen still used to deliver her ironing to my aunt's home at Roseberry, Llandissilio. She said that no one could iron skirts quite as well as Mannie.

Glandŵr was a different place when I was small. It was busy and we even had a few sweet shops. Everything used to come up on the Cardi Bach train – even the hay. I remember collecting medicine for my grandfather from Rhydowen Station, which would have come all the way from Dolycwrt. I would go to see the porter in the station office. He was a kind and understanding gentleman but, having come from England, he could not speak Welsh. So I had to practice my English before going.

We used to have a lot of fun on the station. The cobbler was in a little shed, where he had his own fire. He also had a big jar of sweets – usually mint imperials – so we often called with him. We enjoyed seeing the steam trains arriving, each one bringing more activity to the village, and often returning patients from Dolycwrt Surgery.

Charles Dunford – but known as John – is a native of Whitland, who, as a small child, lived near Dolycwrt. Over the years he remembers many of the doctors, but has a story to tell about Dr Owen, dating back to his younger days:

When I was a boy, Dr Owen was living at Dolycwrt. I used to spend a lot of time near the surgery at the bottom of the meadow by the river. We called it the 'Dingle.' It was an area which flooded, and we did some fishing there. Tom Davies was living in Coedycwrt, next door to the surgery. He was a general handyman for Dr Owen, also his gardener and chauffeur. I was friendly with Tom's son, Basil, and I remember once we all went in the car with Dr Owen, to Sealyham hospital, near Letterston. Tom was driving – slowly as usual – and when we passed the Square in the middle of Haverfordwest, a policeman stopped us.

In those days most traffic went through Castle Square, and there was always a policeman on duty. He stopped us because Tom's small case was on the step of the car. He had forgotten to move it when we set off. I remember Dr Owen being amused about this. He was a kind man, very likeable.

It was around this time that Dr Owen had the assistance of Nurse Owen, who lived in St Mary's Street, fifty yards from the surgery. She spent years in the locality, working hard, covering the district on her bicycle. The late Ivor Evans, a bank manager in Whitland who lived at Brynmelyn, once told me that Nurse Owen gave him a miniature doctor's case when he was a small boy. She had a kind heart and is remembered for her many wonderful deeds – yet she could be firm, too. David Kuhl, formerly of Môr Hafren, North Road, explained:

I had been bitten by a dog when I was going home for dinner one day from school. At the time, a few of us were kicking a ball around, and, when we got below the station gates, the ball rolled away into the station sidings.

This is where coal was stored ready for delivery by hauliers on their horse and carts. Being dinner time, some of the men had disappeared – probably to the pub for a drink – leaving the horse and wagons to be supervised by a couple of dogs.

I remember innocently going in to fetch the ball, and, when I bent down, a dog lunged forward and bit me on the arm.

When I went home to Trevaughan, my arm was bad. My granny called Nurse Owen, and there were no such things as injections for us in those days. I had to have bread poultice in boiling water. This was put on my arm.

I remember Nurse Owen saying, 'Ouch!', because it was warm in her hands. Then she applied it to my arm, and I said, 'Ouch,' too. Then wallop; she gave me a smack.

She used to come to the Council School to inspect our hair to see if we had nits. And if we did, we would be sent home with instructions. There was no messing around with Nurse Owen. She was firm and also fair but everybody used to be petrified of her in the school.

Dr Owen had plenty of variety, even if he did not have a lot of spare time. As the Christmas of 1928 approached he was speaking in the annual prize day of the Whitland County Intermediate School, as Chairman of the Board of Governors. He mentioned that the children who deserved prizes would be rewarded, while praising the education system for giving all children a fair chance. The following is an extract from his speech, which appeared in *The Welshman* of September 14th 1928:

The school had done well during the past year and the results were excellent, and were comparable with any county school of a similar type in the whole country . . . and, with elementary and secondary schools established all over the country bringing to the child in the humble cottage the opportunity of receiving an efficient education, those who had shown intellect had thrived as a result of it.

Now nearing his 44th birthday, and fast approaching his 20th year of service at Dolycwrt, Dr Owen had the opportunity of invaluable assistance. A young man from the locality, who had attended the Whitland County School, and who had recorded great success in his medical examinations, was looking to return to his homeland. He was a determined and ambitious person, who held on to strong principles and standards. He was well connected in the area with family and friends, and a fluent Welsh speaker. More importantly, he had a wonderful sense of feeling for the local characters of the day. He cared greatly about people, and medicine was his world. His homecoming would bring great excitement and, in the spare consulting room at Dolycwrt, a large oak desk awaited his arrival.

Dr Phillip Gibbin FRCS

D R PHILLIP GIBBIN was one of Wales' truest countrymen, having been brought up among the wide open countryside of Login, with all its steep hills and valleys, just five miles north of Whitland. A farmer's son from a large family, he was raised at Pen-yr-Allt farm, where a fast flowing stream passes near the farmhouse on its way to the old mill, before emerging near the Login 'falls' section of the river Taf, amidst the heavy sound of fresh water flow. There it continues, under the pretty stone bridge near the Login halt of the former Cardi Bach line. With all its natural beauty, this Taf valley was once serious railway territory, where its low levels weaved through the hills, like a secret corridor. It was in this natural setting – where the four seasons of the year significantly impact upon the scenery – that Dr Gibbin grew to love the simple ways of country life in his native Wales.

For the young Phillip Gibbin in his early days, schooling could not have provided greater fun or adventure. Sharing the same valley with Pen-yr-Allt, and less than 100 yards upstream, was Pen-y-gaer Local Board School, pitched high-up on the steep wooded bank, like an alpine chalet near a mountain top. This could certainly be the setting for Enid Blyton's *Famous Five* or *Secret Seven* stories and, for this young academic, happy to go orienteering to school on a fine day, this was the size of his task. There could be no greater experience of country education than what Pen-y-gaer School offered Dr Gibbin, and the Log Book[45] entries dating back to Dr Gibbin's time at the school bear testimony to this:

November 13th 1908 . . . this week the master took the upper form along the roadside and gave them a very interesting lesson on trees.

March 19th 1909 . . . gave an interesting lesson on a chaffinch that the children caught in school.

June 30th 1911 . . . lectured on rose growing and bee keeping. Boys seemed very interested. Drew shallots and transplanted sprouts.

In the warmth and homeliness of this natural environment, where the old-fashioned stove kept the cold winter days at bay, Dr Gibbin, in the company of little more than a dozen children, started out on his long journey in education.

There were few cars then and far too many hills to cycle to the County School at Whitland. So this meant that Login children, embarking upon the second stage of their schooling, would meet on the tiny station platform and jump aboard the steam train. Unlike many of his class who stayed in Whitland during the long school weeks, the aspiring doctor usually made the journey back and forth each day, preferring to return home to his family and the farm. This meant an early rise and a sturdy walk, down the steep hill into the tiny village. In the course of his earlier education, there is no doubt that Phillip Gibbin filled his lungs with plenty of healthy fresh air, and this continued after his school days when he took his well-earned place at the University College of Wales, in Aberystwyth.

There, Dolycwrt's future doctor could experience the seri-

45 Carmarthenshire Archives Service.

ous atmosphere of learning and study contained within the sweep of Aberystwyth's stunning sea-front stage. It is there that he immersed himself in science subjects in preparation for his future road to medicine. Enjoying the Welsh culture, abundant use of the native language and a sense of freedom, Dr Gibbin could not ask for more.

After leaving Aberystwyth, he moved onwards to Cardiff, where he did most of his medical studies. He obtained his BSc Wales in 1924, on the way to obtaining the LRCP and MRCS (Eng) qualifications in 1926 when he, no doubt, enjoyed a taste of London's famous medical establishments. Dr Gibbin then undertook a series of appointments, including: Senior Residential Medical Officer at Park Hospital, Flixton; House Surgeon of Caernarvon and Anglesey Infirmary, Bangor; and Senior House Surgeon of Rochdale Infirmary.[46] During this time, he felt the urge to climb one notch further with his studies – striking while the iron was still hot, just like the little blacksmith at Cwm Miles, down the road from his farm in Login.

The next step was to become a Fellow of the Royal College of Surgeons, when, in Edinburgh in 1930, he became one of a small élite group of outstanding medical professionals to record such success. Whilst experiencing life in Scotland's capital, he was, no doubt, reminded about the famous medical events that took place a century earlier when two serial murderers, William Burke and William Hare, provided human bodies for the ambitious anatomy surgeon and lecturer Professor Robert Knox to dissect.[47]

There was great excitement in Dr Gibbin's family with the news of his placement at Dolycwrt. Indeed, Dr Gibbin was re-

---

46 The Royal College of Physicians, Information Centre, *The Medical Directory*.
47 Edinburgh – Royal Mile – Burke and Hare website, as at March 1st 2011.

turning in a blaze of glory, having excelled himself in medical studies. John Davies, today living in Whitland but originally from Brynafon Villa, Login, also attended Pen-y-gaer School, and, in later years got to know Dr Gibbin well. He explained what this new appointment would have meant to Dr Gibbin:

> Dr Gibbin had every reason to be proud of himself. He was from a large family and they had sacrificed a lot for him to go to college. He had brought honour to them by doing so well. Although he was ambitious, Dr Gibbin was also a family man. He looked forward to being with his family again; he was very fond of his Uncle Ben.
>
> In those days, people in Login didn't travel far. The horizon was the limit of their world. Carmarthen was a long way to go then – let alone Edinburgh. Dr Gibbin had become a much-travelled person; he was returning home a different man.
>
> Dolycwrt was well established, serving a wide area all around Dr Gibbin's home countryside. Dr Owen had been there for years and was extremely popular. He would look after his new assistant, helping him onto the medical ladder.
>
> Of course, farming had taught Dr Gibbin all about hard work. He knew that people didn't have money to pay doctors. The average farm worker's wage in the 1930s was around ten shillings per week; times were difficult. But Dr Gibbin was determined, and he knew that things were developing at that time, like cars being available. He would have been full of excitement, raring to go.

Doctors Owen and Gibbin – the County School Old Boys

N OW FULLY SETTLED as a country practitioner at Dol-ycwrt, Dr Gibbin was enjoying himself, helping anyone who dialled 'Whitland 10' for the surgery. Together, he and Dr Owen formed a good team, working well for the good name of the practice. They were seen as two 'old boys' from the County School and were both popular in the town.

Only a couple of months after Dr Gibbin's arrival, he and Dr Owen attended the annual awards ceremony for the ambulance class members. For a number of years, Dr Owen had enjoyed supporting the local Great Western Railway first aid team in this work. The railway men had proved to be dedicated and talented students, having won all manner of regional and national competitions over the years. Of course, Dr Owen, had always been comforted knowing that immense first-aid expertise existed in the town, especially when he was away in distant corners of the Practice. The event, held at the Grosvenor Hotel, was recorded in the *Pembroke County and West Wales Guardian* on March 25th 1932:

> Dr Gibbin, in his opening remarks, thanked the railway-men for inviting him and said that he had always been interested in first aid work. Ambulance work was charita-ble work and it meant giving up a great deal of time. The awards he was about to present were the emblems of the spirit of sacrifice.

Dr Owen appealed to the older ambulance workers to attend the classes, and to assist the younger members in gaining knowledge of first aid work. He hoped that the meeting would be an incentive to the employees of the G.W.R. to take to first aid work. He stressed the value of ambulance workers to the community.

On the social scene, Dr Owen would have known about the football matches taking place over the road from Dolycwrt at the Recreation Field. The 'O'Connor's Cup', named after Cecil O'Connor, a local sports enthusiast, who used to run both a nursery and florist's shop in town, was a much sought-after prize. Local players entered the tournament, lining up for such teams as the tradesmen, clerks, publicans, G.W.R., milk factory, or even the 'Casuals', this latter team being comprised of individuals who didn't fit into the other teams, or were not, perhaps, chosen. One of these matches is recorded in *The Welshman* on May 5th 1933 – the reporter cleverly adding to the occasion:

> There was considerable excitement on the Recreation ground on Saturday evening when the G.W.R. soccer eleven met the Casuals in their round of the O'Connor's Cup. The ground was in good condition, except that the goalmouths were rather wet. It is to be feared that the water in the goalmouth at the Memorial Hall end cost the Casuals the game, for their goalkeeper (and who would blame him?) preferred to stand outside the pool with the result that he was twice beaten by dropping shots, which he might have saved had he stood on his own line.

In this same popular paper on March 9th 1934, was a report of the Whitland Angling Club's annual dinner at the Yelverton Hotel. This was a night of great humour and leg-pulling among the speakers, and it was very much a doctor's night, too, with Dr Hugh Philipps of Clyngwynne, a country doctor in Llanboidy, who later did locum work at Dolycwrt, Dr Gibbin and Dr Rowley Thomas present. A short extract of the interchange between Dr Gibbin – proposing a toast to the Towy Fishery Board – and Dr Rowley Thomas, who responded, is as follows:

> Dr Gibbin said that the Board included several important members – also Dr Rowley Thomas, who was a big noise (laughter). He (the speaker) had known him for many years and had listened to his yarns with amazement. The Board represented voluntary service, and had been in existence over fifty years, safeguarding and protecting the interests of the fishermen. It prevented the monopoly of a few by giving rights to all men alike.

Dr Thomas, of Parke farm, who was also a Councillor, responded, addressing the gathering as 'Fellow Poachers':

> He thanked the Proposer for his kind remarks and did not propose to contradict him (laughter). He had taken on a public job and expected bricks, as long as those bricks were not thrown too hard.

One of the games that Dr Gibbin enjoyed at that time was quoits. This involved throwing a heavy flat ring of iron, circular in shape and similar in size to a horse shoe, whilst aiming for a peg some 18 – 21 yards away. Quoits came in different weights, and whilst the idea sounds straight forward, in practice it was not. At this time, quoits was extremely popular in Whitland and in the neighbouring country villages, especially with the farmers. Howard Gibbon is pleased to explain its origin:

All of that started back in the days of the horse and cart. A farmer would send his servant boy to a farrier with a horse to be shoed. Often he would meet another boy in the same situation, and they would pick up the old shoes and throw them at some distant object. They developed this into a competition then. A large sleeper would be cut in half to make a box, and it was filled with clay. Then a peg was placed in the middle of it. Quoits were round and heavy, and there was an art to the game. To be a good thrower you had to have a lot of practice.

As a rule, quoits matches were held alongside some other agricultural event, such as a farm show. When sheep shearing took place in the 'Fisher's Field' behind the pub, in the 1930s, there would always be people playing, whilst others went over to watch. Of course, Dr Gibbin enjoyed the social occasions, especially the farming scene, so it is understandable that he got involved with quoits.

Both Dr Gibbin and Dr Owen would have known about another competition taking place around this time: making a scarecrow. My father was keen to do well, and had help from a mason and a carpenter to carve-out a face. On its head was a German helmet and a muzzle-loaded gun was in its hands. This entry won the prize and it was exhibited across the road from Dolycwrt in the Council School yard. It was quite a talking point at the time, and the doctors would have seen it from the surgery driveway.

Songs of the Valley and a Sad Farewell

D R OWEN, who had often voiced his concerns about out-
dated medical facilities, was thrilled to hear news that
a new purpose-built isolation hospital for Carmarthenshire
was opening at Tumble, Llanelli. This would accommodate
sufferers of diphtheria and scarlet fever, and it is where his
patients, too, would be referred. At a time when the days of the
workhouse at Narberth had come to an end – and medicine's
momentum was sailing onwards beyond the quarantine boats
of old – better days clearly lay ahead. Dr Owen would have
been equally pleased to hear that there were to be additional
district nurses allocated to the area. This would be music to
his ears.

Of course, doctors had their own opinions on the endless
medicinal remedies that were advertised regularly in the
newspapers. Some of the old cures, such as honey and lemon,
were popular, while the virtues of a stiff whiskey, or a drop
of brandy, also continued to cure more than the odd sniffle
or cold. But the medicines that Doctors Owen and Gibbin
dispensed carried their individual trademark. Their mixtures
were personal and, although sometimes remembered for
having plenty of sediment or a ghastly taste, they were always
gratefully accepted. Indeed, many patients believed that
possessing a bottle of the doctors' prescribed medicine was
more important than the actual contents of the mixture.

Dr Owen and Dr Gibbin also recognised the positive
nature of another therapy – if not a cure – that was readily

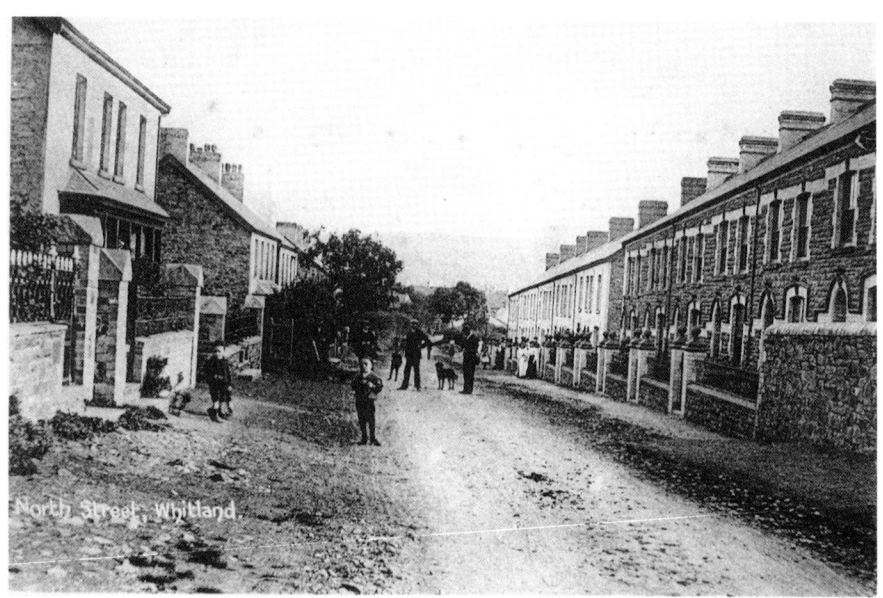

North Road, Whitland before the arrival of the motor car.
Anne Bowen's collection

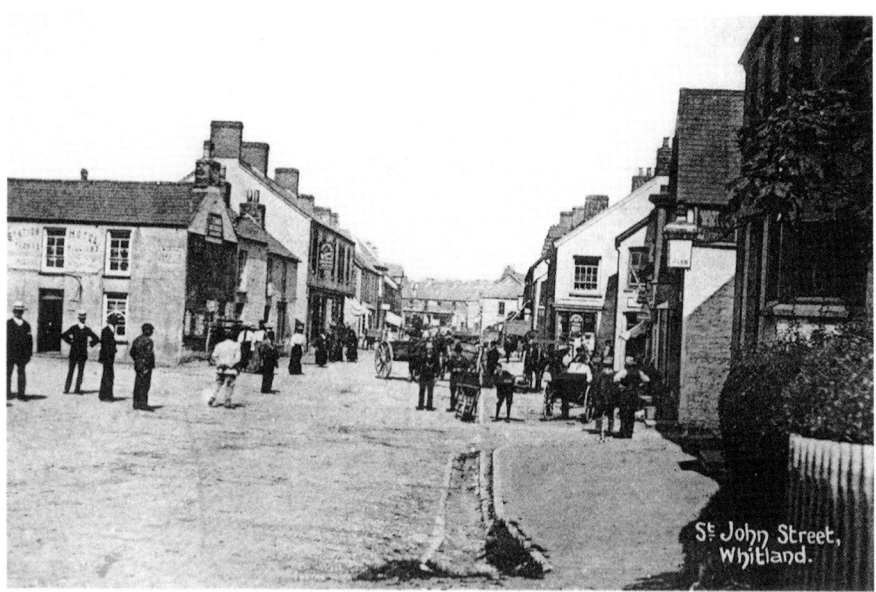

St John Street, Whitland; a fashionable place for shopping!
Anne Bowen's collection

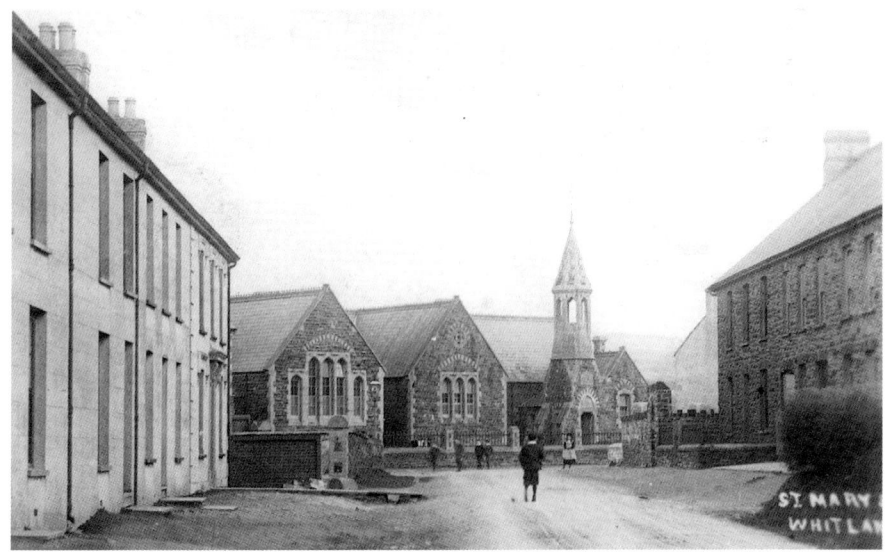

St Mary's Street, Whitland. Dolycwrt stands at the end of the street on the right hand side.
Anne Bowen's collection

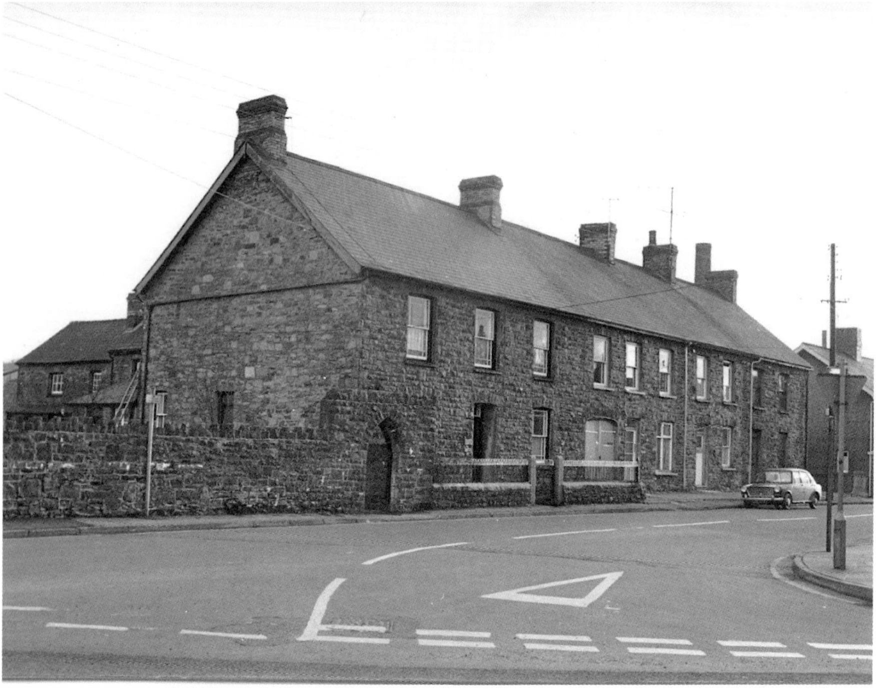

Dolycwrt as part of a terrace of houses in the early 1970s.
W. Rainbow's collection

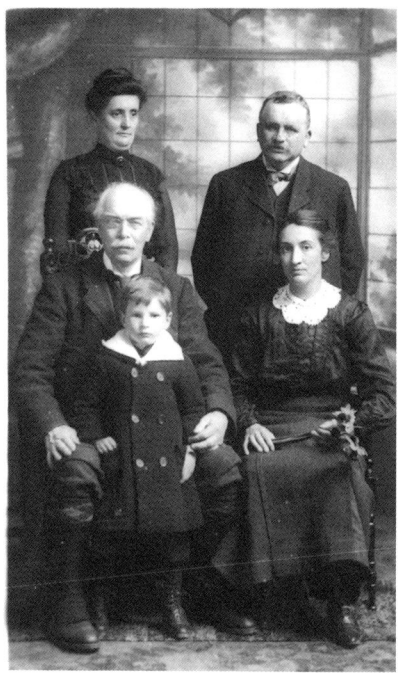

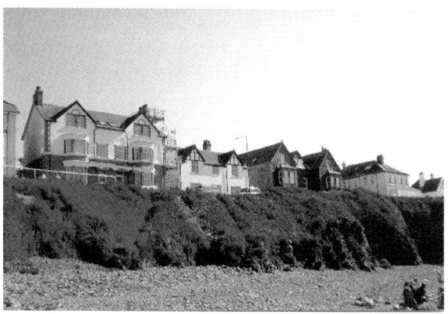

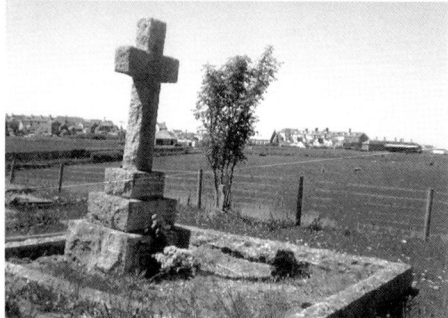

Dr and Mrs Creswick Williams, standing.
Dr and Mrs Bowen-Jones, seated
Mrs C. Rees-Davies' collection

The homes of Dr and Mrs Creswick Williams,
in Borth: Bay Ridge Villa (extreme left) and
Cliff Haven (large house on extreme right).
And their last resting place at Borth cemetary.

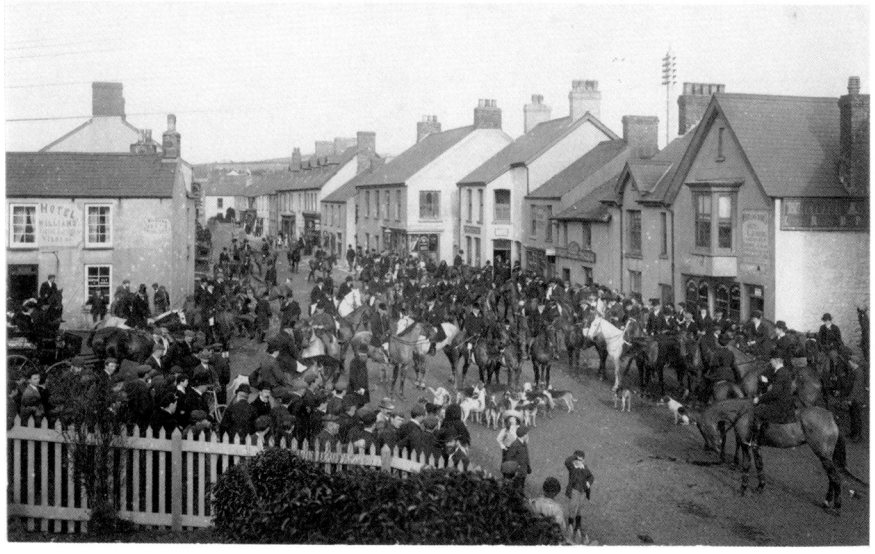

The Hunt scene in Whitland. Many a patient kept the Dolycwrt doctors busy when they fell
off their horse.
Carmarthenshire Archives Service

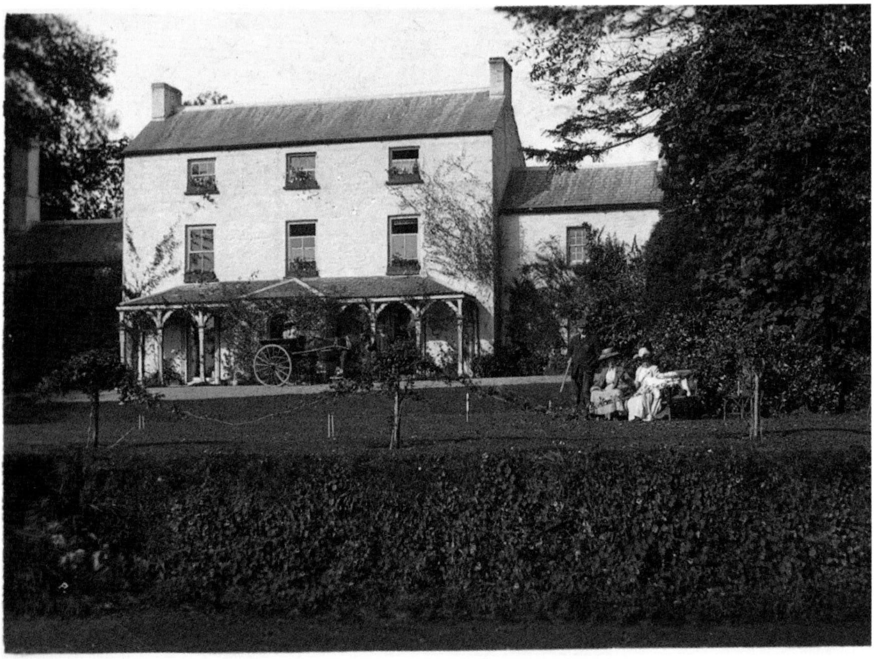

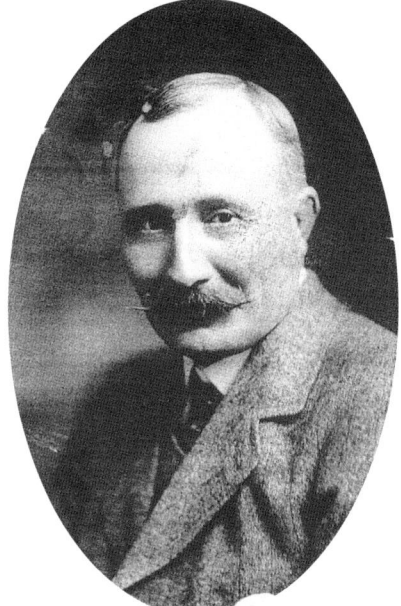

Parke Farm, Henllan Amgoed, the former home of Dr Rowley Thomas.
His old surgery is on the right.
Mrs Olga Roberts' collection

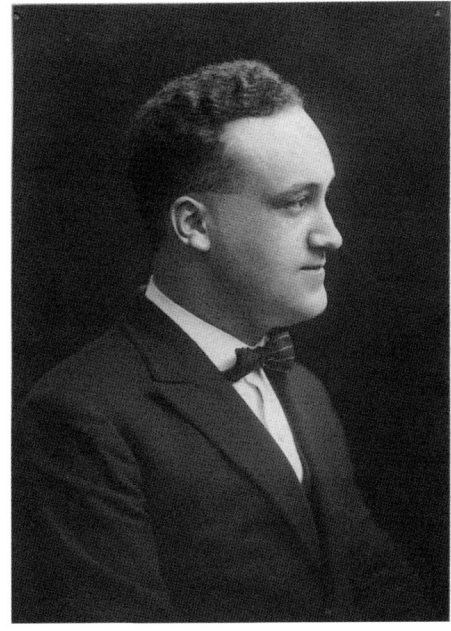

Dr Rowley Thomas
Gerwyn Williams' collection

Dr Phillip Gibbin

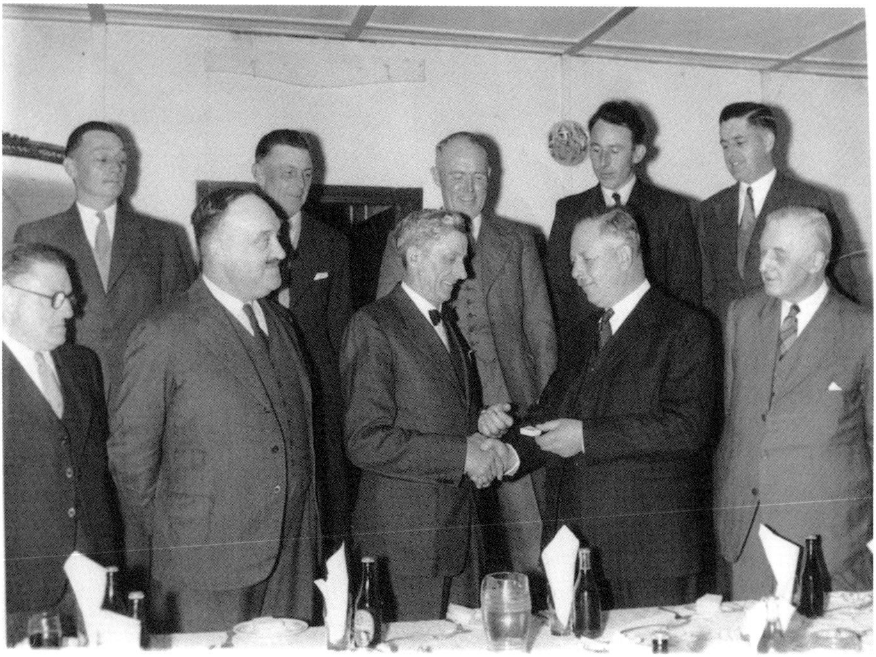

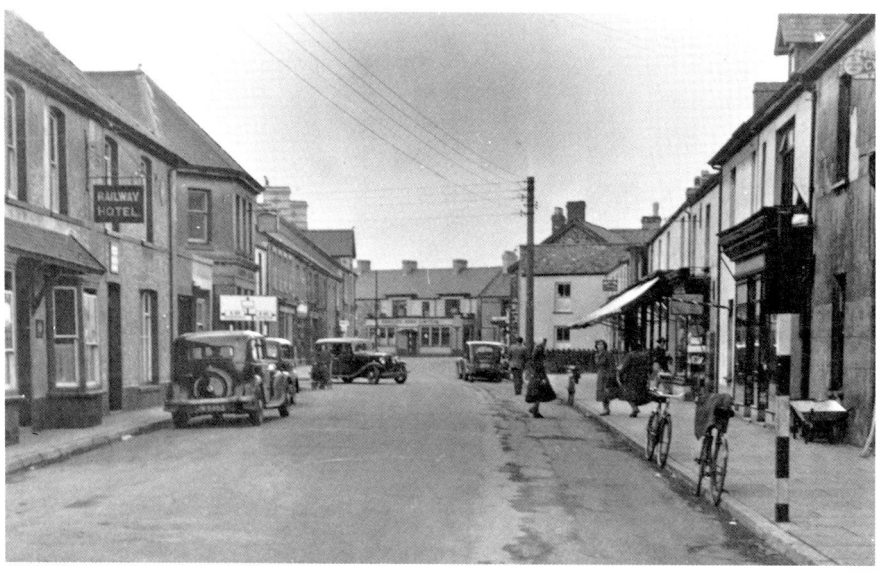

Dr Phillip Gibbin at a presentation ceremony in Whitland.

A Whitland scene that Dr Phillip Gibbin would be very familiar with.
Carmarthenshire Archives Service

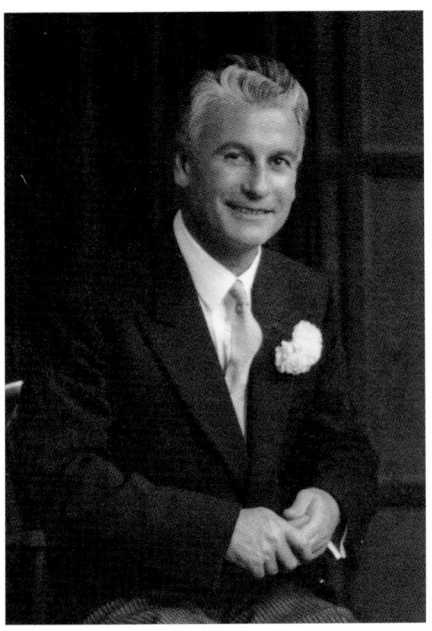

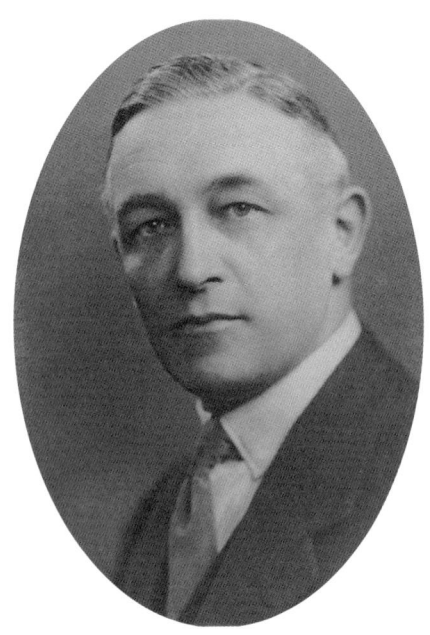

Dr Hirwaun Thomas
Mrs Thomas' collection

Dr William David Owen
Mr John Dyer's collection

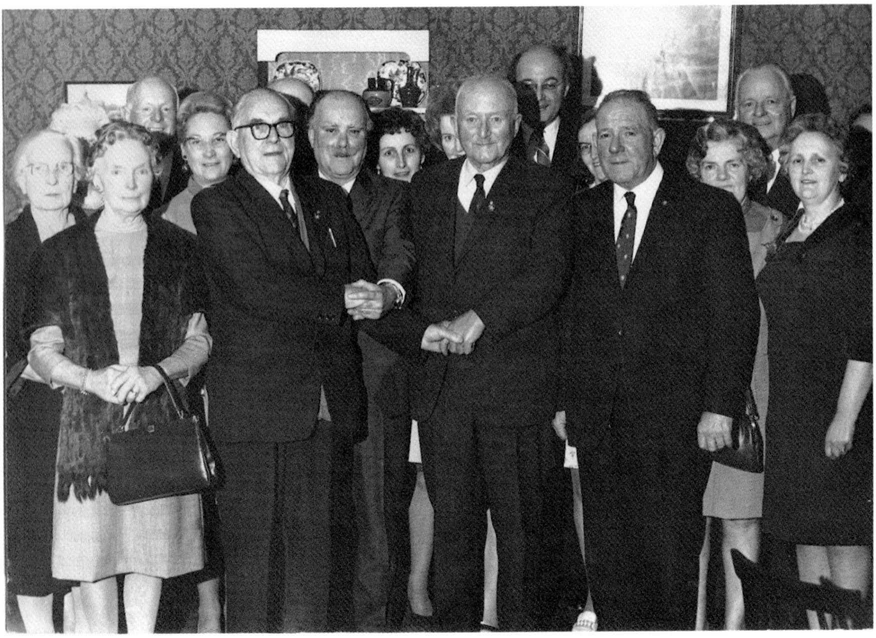

Dr Hugh Lewis-Philipps can be seen just right of centre, with Dr Penn behind him in the back row.

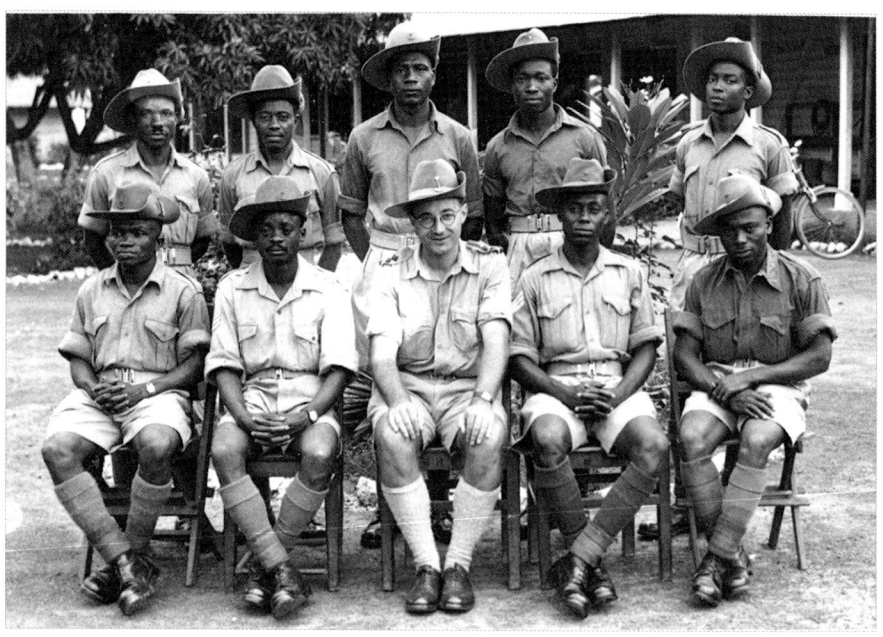

Dr Penn on duty in Nigeria with the 2nd Batallion of the Nigerian Regiment.

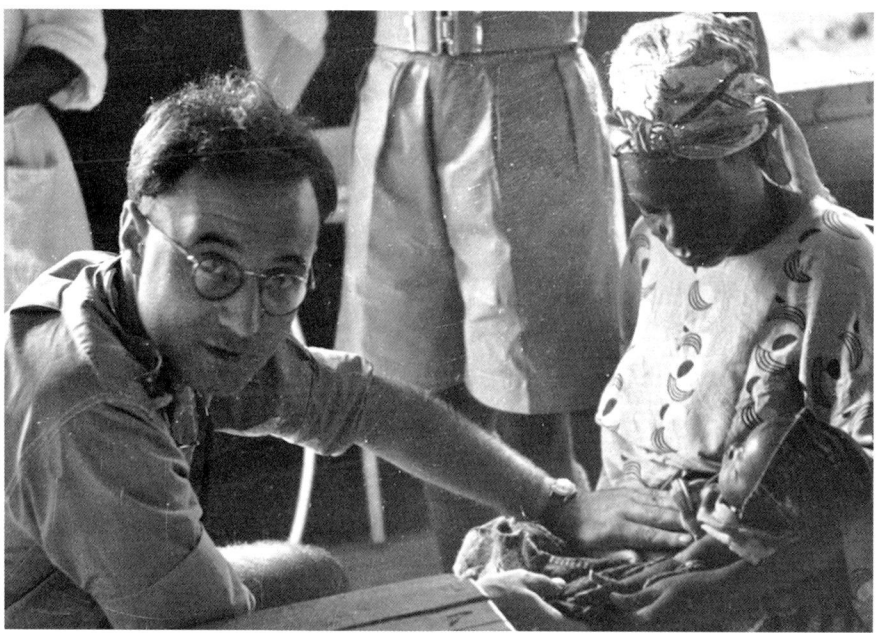

Dr Penn, the Regimental Medical Officer, treating a sick child in Nigeria.

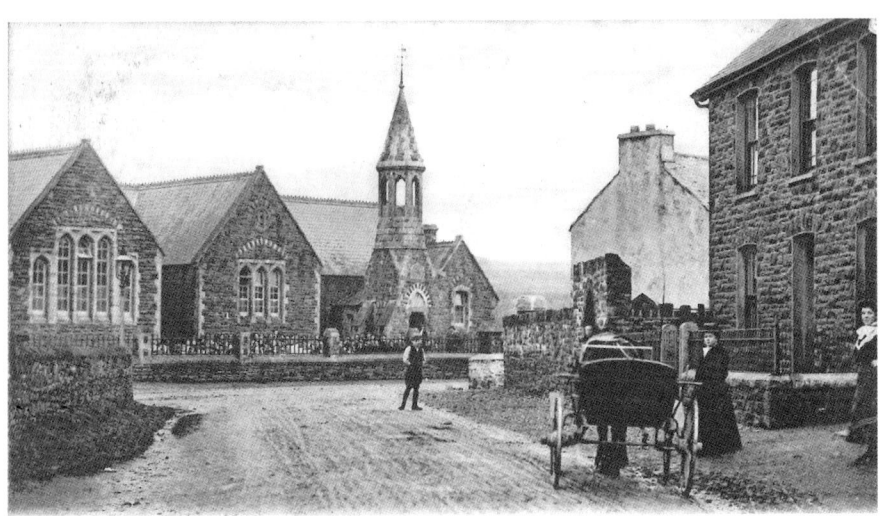

Outside Dolycwrt during the days of Dr Creswick Williams, with the Council School (today's Whitland Primary School) in the background.
Carmarthenshire Archives Service

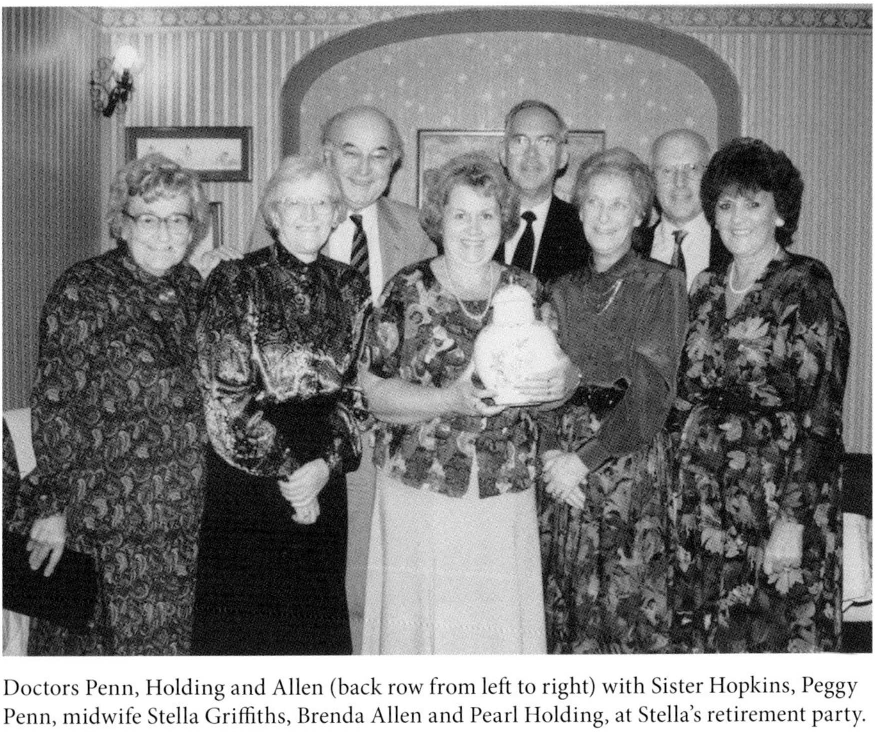

Doctors Penn, Holding and Allen (back row from left to right) with Sister Hopkins, Peggy Penn, midwife Stella Griffiths, Brenda Allen and Pearl Holding, at Stella's retirement party.

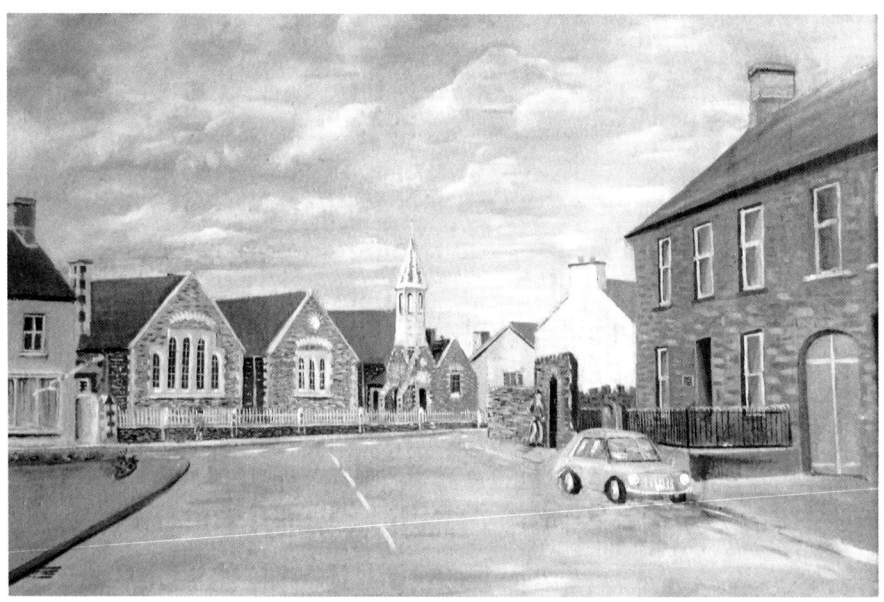

A painting by W. J. Auker which had pride of place on the surgery wall of Dolycwrt for many years. *Plus ça change ...!*

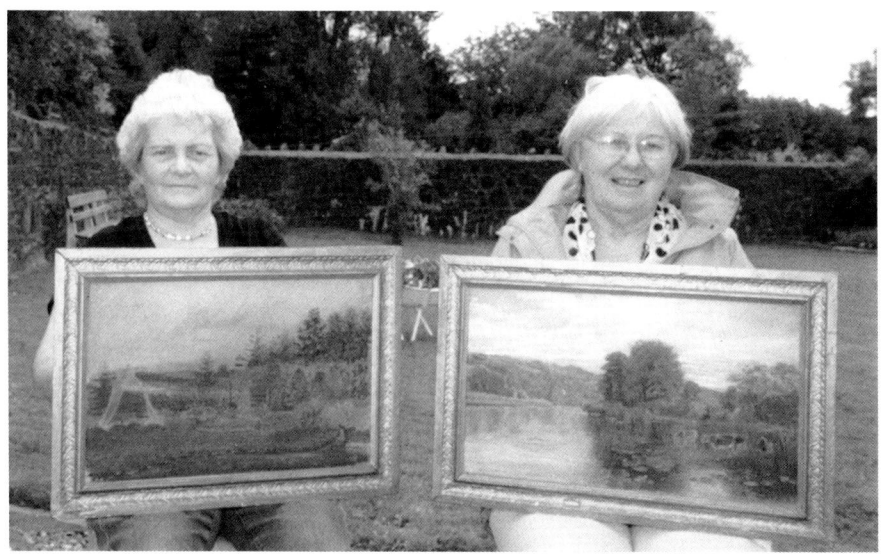

June George and Yvonne Evans with paintings given to their grandmother by Dr and Mrs Creswick Williams. The paintings show an early morning scene at the bottom of the garden by the river Gronw, and the flooded river Gronw in Llanboidy.

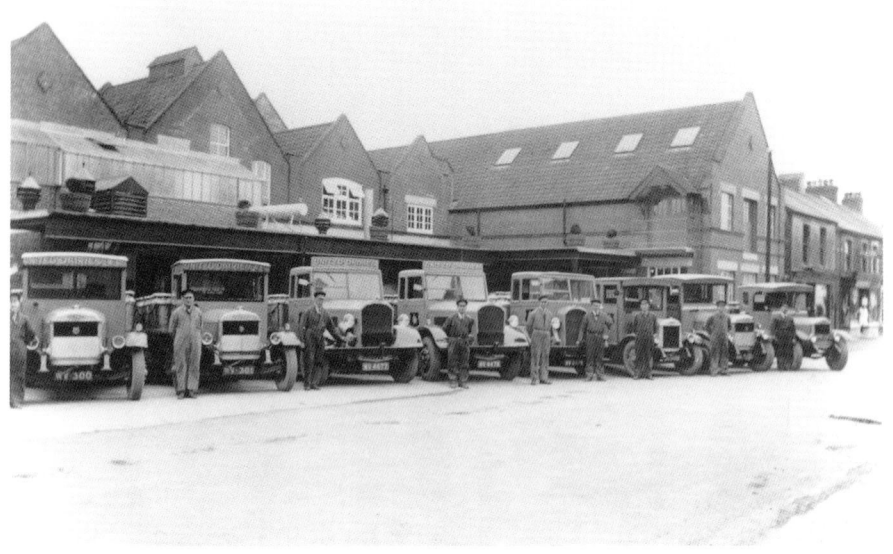

The once mighty United Dairies lorries line up next door to Dolycwrt.
Mr Keith Thomas' collection

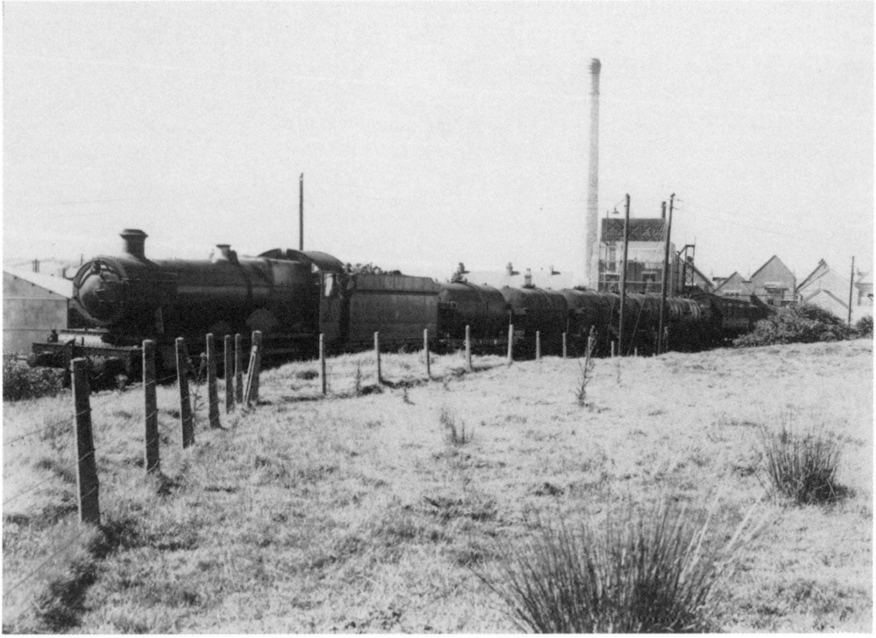

The steam Milk Train, in all its glory, leaves Whitland.
Mr Keith Thomas' collection

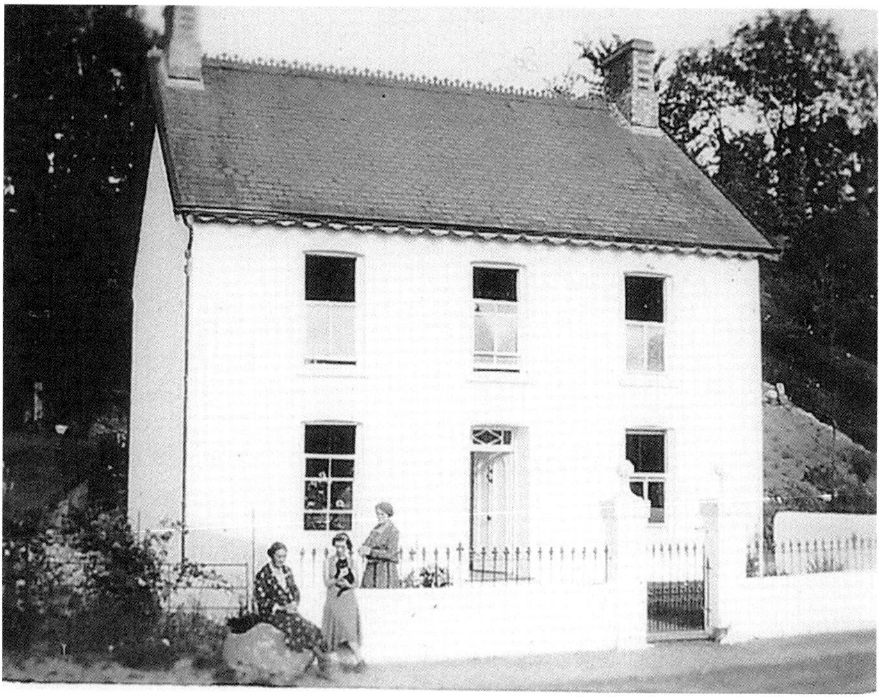

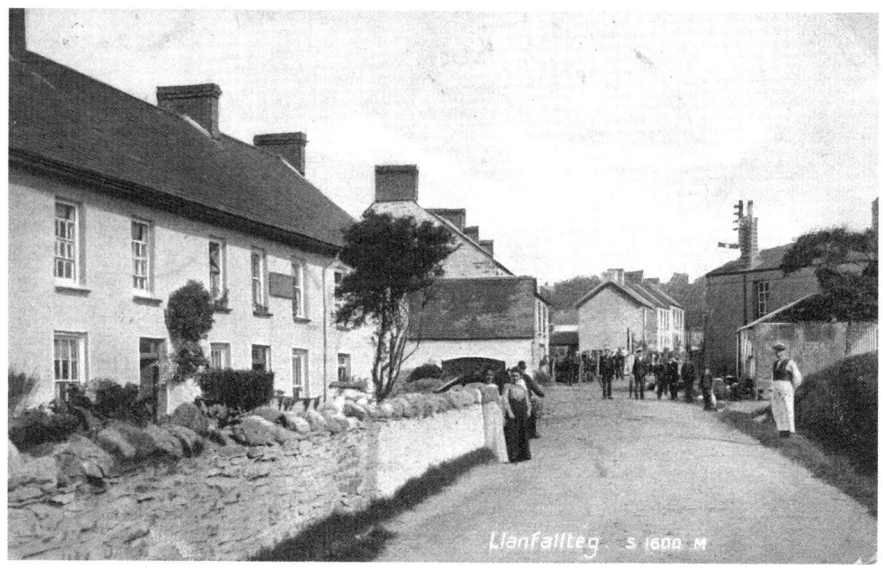

Caroline Rees-Davies outside her home, Glan-yr-Afon, Llanboidy; also the surgery of her father, Dr Bowen-Jones.
Mrs C. Rees-Davies' collection

Llanfallteg, on the Cardi Bach line, where Dr Owen used to hold a Country Surgery.
In the late Willie Reynolds' collection

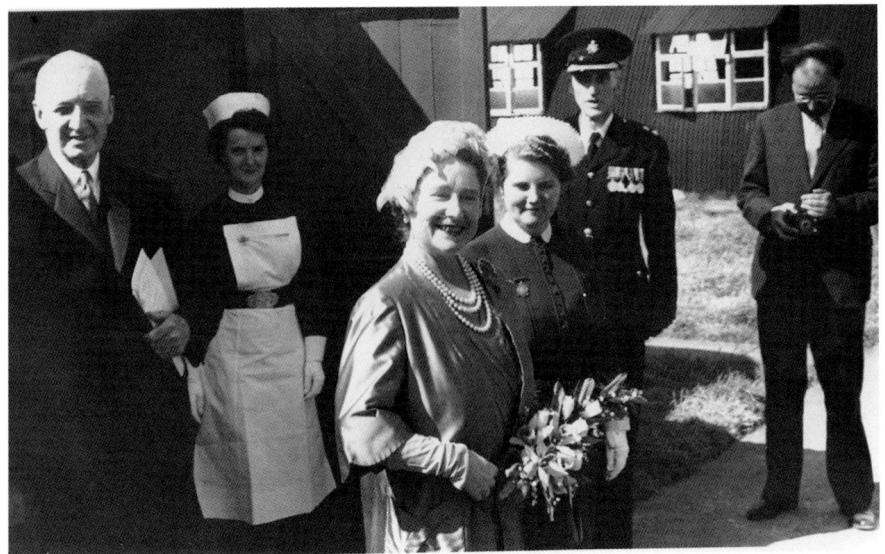

The Queen Mother opens Glangwili Hospital in 1959. Dr Penn can be seen on the extreme right looking into his camera. Note the Nissen huts in the background.

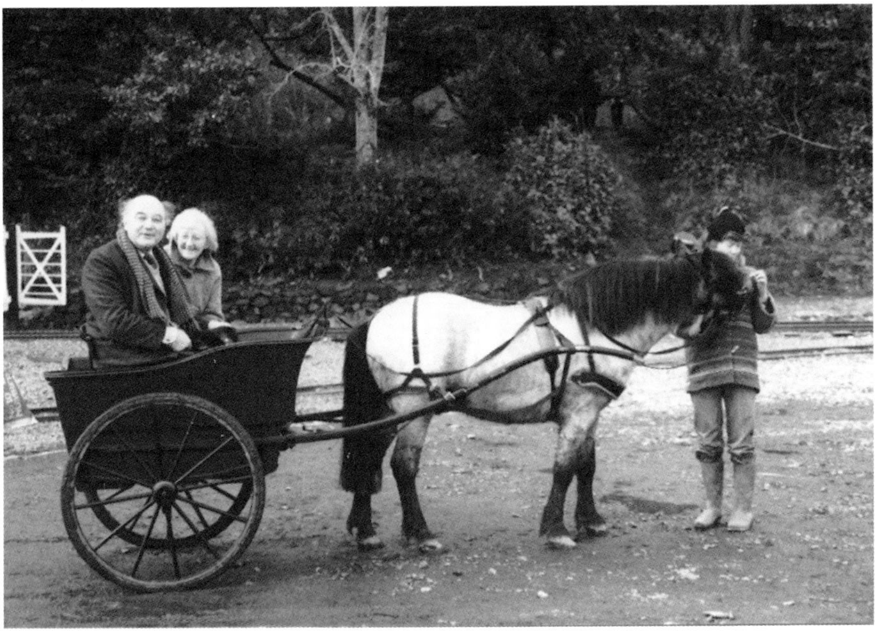

How it might have been in another era . . . a fleet of horse and carts?

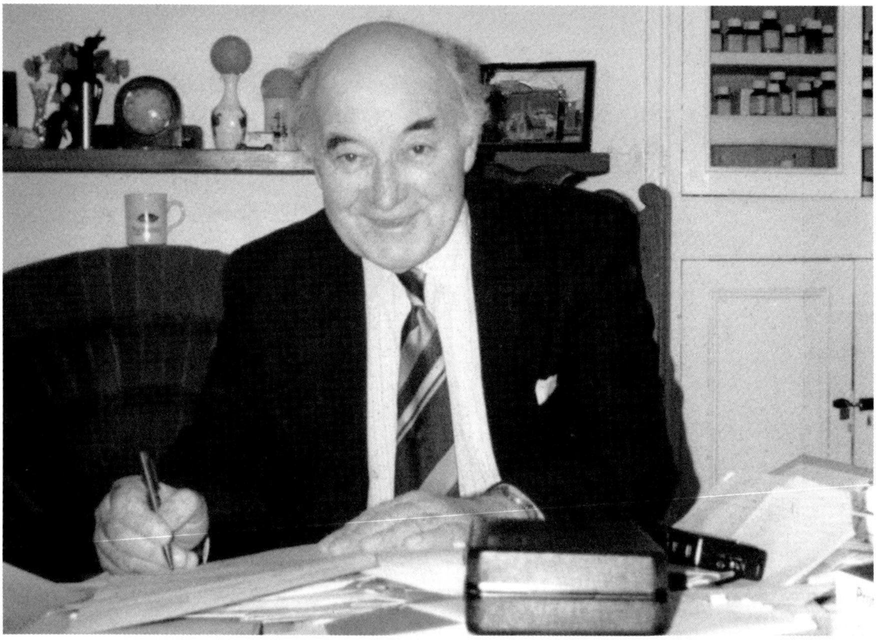

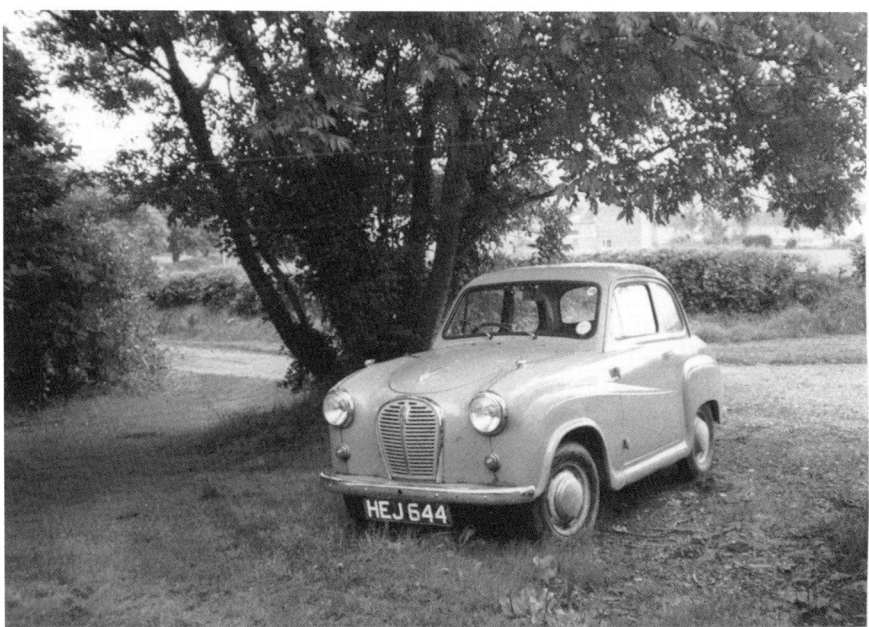

Dr Penn at his desk in Dolycwrt.

One of Dr Penn's fleet of many cars . . . a favourite Austin A35.

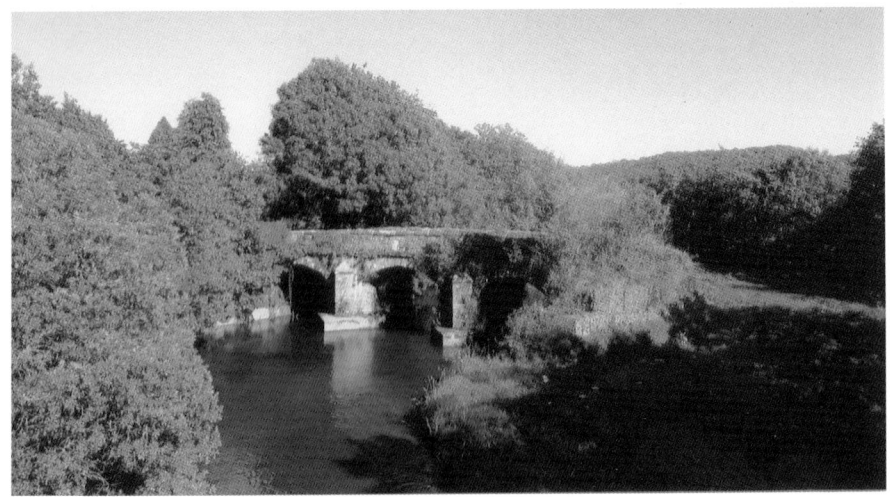

Trevaughan Bridge. The scene of repeated Rebecca Riots and the focus of one of Dr Penn's campaigns.

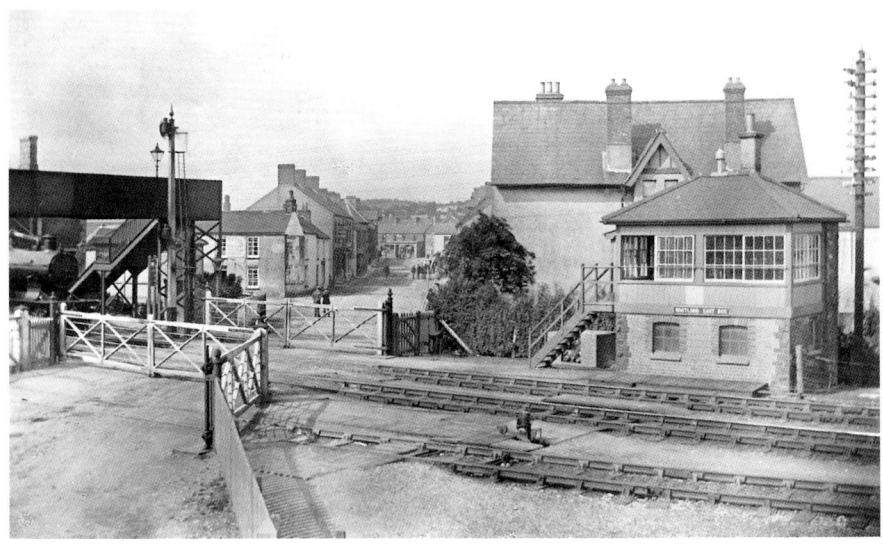

The level crossing and East Box at Whitland, with the Station Hotel in the background.
Carmarthenshire Archives Service

PARC DR. OWEN, WHITLAND
☆

FESTIVAL WEEK

☆

Saturday, August 29th to Sunday, September 6th

President : Dr. MELBOURNE THOMAS

SATURDAY, AUGUST 29th—

BRIGHTER CRICKET

SIX-A-SIDE KNOCK-OUT COMPETITION

ASHGROVE CRICKET GROUND

ADMISSION 1/-

WICKETS PITCHED 2.30 p.m.

☆

SUNDAY, AUGUST 30th—

Grand Celebrity Concert

WHITLAND MALE VOICE CHOIR

GRAMMAR SCHOOL ASSEMBLY HALL

COMMENCING 8 P.M.   ADMISSION 2/6

Guest Artistes :

MISS LORNA IRVING, Member of Guildhall School of Music, London, International, National Blue Ribbon Winner.

WILLIAM MATHIAS, B.Mus., L.R.A.M., Music Lecturer, Bangor University.

...THIAS, L.R.A.M.

...ENS

PARC DR. OWEN DEVELOPMENT COMMITTEE, WHITLAND

PRESENT

5th WHITLAND WEEK 1968

Saturday, 24th August—Sunday, September 1st

President : Mr. Haydn Lewis

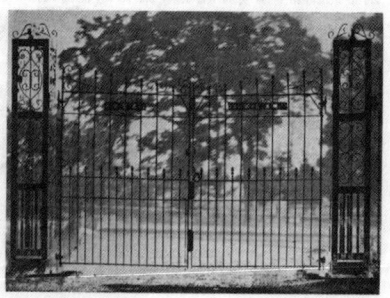

The week's programme
price 1/6

52

Keep your programme—yours may have the lucky number. Prize £2.

Parc Dr. Owen Development Committee hope that the week's ... will bring much pleasure and at the same time help a good cause.

NATIONAL HEALTH SERVICE ACT, 1946.

PEMBROKESHIRE EXECUTIVE COUNCIL.

W. C. SCOURFIELD,
Clerk of the Council.

13, GOAT STREET,
HAVERFORDWEST.
31st December, 1959.

Dear Sir/Madam,

I have to inform you that in consequence of the death of Dr. P. Gibbin of Whitland, your name has been transferred from his list of National Health Service patients to the list of his successor, Dr. G. K. Penn, who will practise at Dolycwrt, Whitland, in partnership with Dr. J. E. Merrell.

If you do not wish your name to remain on Dr. Penn's list you may secure an immediate transfer by presenting your medical card to another doctor for acceptance or by notifying the Council within fourteen days of the receipt of this notice that you object to the transfer. Any request for a transfer received after this period will require prior notice of fourteen days.

Yours faithfully,

W. C. SCOURFIELD.

The Venerable Order of the Hospital of St. John of Jerusalem

FORM W/5

Priory for Wales

Authority is hereby given to Dr. Penn

... to conduct an Examination in First Aid

at Whitland,

(Railway Station).

Estimated Number of Candidates : Men 36 Women —

on 9th March, 1960, at o'clock.

LOCAL HON. SECRETARY :

R. R. P. Rate, Esq.,
Yard Masters Office,
British Railways,
Swansea,
Glam.

NEAREST RAILWAY STATION : Swansea, Glam.

This should be kept by

Principal Secretary.

A flurry of professional and community activities at Whitland, and Dolycwrt was at the heart of it.

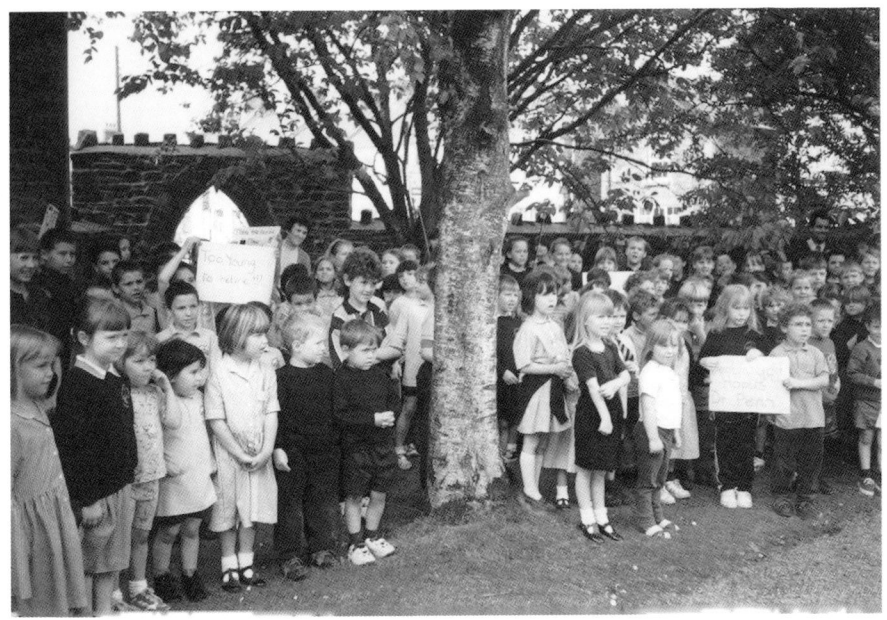

The local primary school children entertain Dr Penn on his last day at Dolycwrt before retiring. The posters read: 'Too young to retire!' and 'Penblwydd hapus, Dr Penn!'

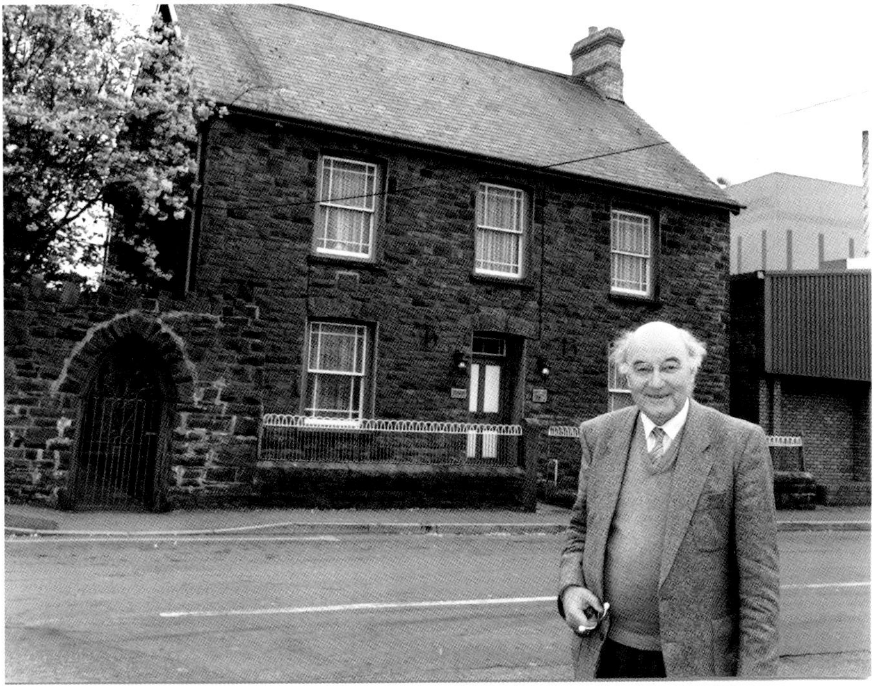

Dr Penn's pride and joy, Dolycwrt, a doctor's surgery for one hundred years.

obtainable in the Taf valley. It did not come in bottles, and it could not be dispensed, but it had played a big part in raising people's spirits and morale for many years. It concerned the regular musicals, concerts, singing festivals, choral events and Cymanfa Ganu gatherings that enriched everybody's lives, and the wealth of talented singers and musicians that made all this possible.

The male voice choir was well-known for having co-ordinated the strong voices of our valley into stirring award-winning performances for many years. As one of the longest serving organisations in the town today, the Whitland Male Voice Choir is often associated with its former long serving conductor, the late Daniel Luther Stephens MBE (Danny). He gave years of dedication – and so did his wife, Mabel, as accompanist – and everyone was thrilled when Danny received Royal recognition. Before him was Tom Davies, who was described many years later in a 50th anniversary booklet *Whitland and District Male Choir 1922 – 1972* (which appears to chart the times of Danny Stephens onwards) as:

a local tailor, of Greenfield House. He was the precentor of music at Tabernacle Congregational Chapel for a long period of years.

Indeed, the combined era of Danny and Tom seem to link almost all the Dolycwrt doctors who participated in the surgery's full century of years, whilst one of these doctors was later to become a singing member. Of course, Dr Owen and Dr Gibbin were never far away from these musical performances, often chairing concerts as well as dances in the town, whilst ensuring that the correct mixtures and tonics kept the vocal chords of their singing patients in tip-top condition.

It was during this same year, 1932, that a 'Grand Performance' of Handel's *Messiah* was presented by the Whitland

Choral Society, at Whitland Town Hall. The programme, costing 2d, and printed by Caxton Works, Whitland, stated that reserved seats were priced at 2/4, 3/6 and 5/-. That evening the soprano, contralto, tenor, and bass artists travelled from London, Treorchy, Merthyr and Nantymoel respectively. As far as the two doctors were concerned, such an outstanding event worked wonders for the patients of their practice. It would send people home with a spring in their steps, whistling on their way to work, and humming their favourite tunes throughout the day.

The following year, a jazz band entertained the crowds at the Whitland carnival, organised to raise money for the Memorial Hall. Whether the doctors crossed the road from Dolycwrt that day is not known, but they were now involved socially with virtually all events in the town. Dr Gibbin had, by now, become president of the quoits club, and Dr Owen had also accepted the presidency of the newly formed town hockey team.

One of Dr Owen's favourite patients was Nancy Davies, who today lives at Tŷ Newydd, Cwmfelin Boeth, overlooking the old flour and grain mill where her late husband, Wil, a member and soloist for the choir for forty years, used to work. As a young girl growing up in a community that excelled in music, Nancy became a talented musician herself, Indeed, she was the organist at Bryn Sion Chapel for thirty-five years, and remembers with fondness the old concerts and services when the chapel was full. Nancy explained the time she visited Dr Owen, way back, in April 1937:

> We had this vicious cockerel on the farm. He was horrible and dangerous, and I got so wild with him one day that I chased him. I was eighteen years old and it was Easter and the demon cockerel, a Rhode Island Red, led me towards

the hayshed. There was an iron girder protruding from the shed, which I didn't see, and I had quite a nasty cut to my head. I chanced it to go down to the surgery because it was Good Friday – 'Grand Dad, please take me down to Doly-cwrt,' I asked.

Mrs Owen opened the front door, and coming up the corridor was her husband, Dr Owen. 'Come in Nancy, what have you been doing?' were his words. Immediately I felt better. There and then, he sat me down in the front room and stitched my wound. He was sorry about the gash I had, because it was nasty, but he was thoroughly amused about the cockerel. He was a treasure to know.

Those kind words from Nancy would be echoed everywhere around the practice. Dr Owen stood out like a beacon and, having devoted himself to Dolycwrt and the local scene since 1913, he was now loved and respected by everyone. Whitland was his world; and with Dr Gibbin's help – and Tom Davies, his friend and next-door neighbour to chauffeur him – his future would surely be bright. But news had been released that Dr Owen was unwell. He had been taken ill at Easter and everybody had been saddened. The announcement that followed a few weeks later was to stun people to silence and to physically shake a whole community. He had died, aged just 48; his journey had come to an end. His work was done, and Nancy had been his last patient.

In Whitland, Login, and Llanglydwen, and in every village or hamlet of the practice, it was as if the lights had gone out. Intense sadness prevailed as Dr Owen's passing seemed to flood the valleys with tears. The local papers rearranged their columns to make room for one of the biggest funerals that Whitland had ever seen.

On Thursday 29th April 1937, shortly before 2.30 in the

afternoon the funeral cortège left the courtyard of Dolycwrt and headed slowly down the narrow driveway. Across the road, in the Council School, the teachers and pupils were paying their own tributes. So often in the past, Dr Owen had entered the beautiful building beneath the bell tower during times of sickness and accidents.[48] This same setting had also seen him preside over many social events and meetings, particularly the welcome-home parties for the war heroes. This day the school would honour him. Every child stood to attention. Not a word, not a gesture, they stood still, as if they were standing in ceremony. Les Rowlands, a local railwayman, remembers the occasion well, because he stood so still that he fainted. Miss Lucy Walters, the popular teacher, revived him with cold water.

Up the road, in Soar Chapel was a sea of faces, all sad and tearful that day, but all with treasured memories of their friend, the doctor. Patients had travelled from the countryside to be there for him – and Dr Gibbin was an honoured bearer. The small funeral leaflet, which had black braiding around its edge, simply said in Welsh, 'Funeral Service of the late, Dr William David Owen'. Inside were the hymns *Paham yr wylwn am y rhai* (Why for those we grieve?) and *Beth sydd i mi yn y byd* (What is there for me in this world?). There is something about a Welsh hymn that stirs the heart, indeed the singing comes from the heart; certainly it did that day. Amidst the crowds of people, the many tributes, the bounteous flowers and all the tears, Dr Owen was laid to rest. Dr Owen's nephew David Morris, told me:

> Uncle 'Dick' was always so good to people, and, in his gen-
> erosity, he did so many great deeds. I know for a fact, that

---

48 Whitland Primary School Log Book.

he helped people who could not pay their rents or their bills. With him, there were no limits to his kindnesses.

David's sister Kay, said,

> I found an old book belonging to Uncle Dick recording his movements and visits. Written at the end of each column were the words 'No Charge'. I don't think he ever charged.

In the coming months, three memorable words appeared on Dr Owen's tombstone as the perfect epitaph – *the Beloved Physician.*

Dolycwrt in the Grip of War

THE SAD SCENES in Soar Chapel left an unforgettable impression in Dr Gibbin's mind. That day patients climbed aboard the early Cardi Bach train from the outlying villages of the practice to pay their respects. It was all very sorrowful, touching and tragic but life had to go on. Seizing the reins of Dolycwrt, Dr Gibbin made sure that the little surgery and all its patients were in safe hands. There would be no backward steps with him. This was a matter of heritage; it was a matter of honour, too. Dolycwrt would, most certainly, move on.

Sadly, so also would the Germans. War was drawing closer now; feelings were running high. It is understandable that there was tension in the air when a large band of British Legion members reported to the Memorial Hall, Whitland, a few months later to hear the chairman's stern address. Reverend W. J. Bowen stated in *The Welshman*:

> There is not an ex-serviceman whatever his physical disability, resultant upon his war experience, who does not feel justifiably proud of the fact that he exhibited his love for his Motherland, his love for her glorious traditions, music and language . . . What hundreds of our fallen comrades prayed for with their dying breath was a united Britain and a united world.

The British Legion was now active, strong and robust, across the country – and Britain needed this. When the annual dinner of the Whitland and District Branch was held in the early months of 1939, we know from reports in *The Welshman* that Dr Gibbin was one of three doctors present. They were all men of stature and good speakers, too. But, that night, in the cosy environment of the Lamb Inn, Llanboidy, each had another role to play as the nation hardened its resolve. They took their turn: Dr Hugh Lewis-Philipps, a former Wimbledon tennis player; Dr Rowley Thomas, a former Welsh rugby international; and Dr Gibbin, a Fellow of the Royal College of Surgeons. They were all winners in their own right; now, behind their words of praise for the British Legion movement was a thread of steel, because the country and the locality needed leaders from every walk of life.

Leonard Coleman – drafted into Whitland some years earlier to manage the growing milk factory – was one of these. He had come from Chewton Mendip as a highly respected cheese expert, and now shared with Dr Gibbin the health concerns of his expanding workforce. Often seen passing Dolycwrt on his way to work, he was behind every moving function in this now vast enterprise, which was still spreading its boundaries within the town. As a survivor of the Great War, he knew the measurements of the enemy, too, and his military experience was vital to the town.

Another was Major Godfrey Evan Schaw Protheroe-Beynon DL, JP, of Trewern Mansion. He had a medical background, being the son of a surgeon-general and, in 1907, he was High Sheriff of Carmarthenshire.[49] He fought in the Great War with distinction, where he attained his rank. He knew that troubles lay ahead. Technology had progressed to such an extent that air bombing raids, incendiary devices and gas explosions could wreak havoc. This could impact enormously on Dr Gibbin and his medical colleagues. Everybody had to

---

49 The *Carmarthen Journal*, 14 November, 1958, Carmarthen Library.

be prepared because enormous changes lay ahead.

In the summer months of 1939 – still peacetime, but only just – a new doctor arrived in Dolycwrt. Dr Gwynne Morris Evans, from Burry Port, was replacing Dr Mansel Williams, a native of north Wales, who was leaving after a year spent assisting Dr Gibbin. Dr Evans had barely used his stethoscope when Germany invaded Poland. The waiting was over; here was wretched warfare once again. It was time to brace one's self for action, as both Whitland and Dolycwrt responded to wartime rules. John Llewellyn, mentioned earlier, describing his father's return from war, explained:

> Across the country, everyone had Air Raid Protection committees. There would be divisional wardens and district wardens, and it was imperative that the same strict new practices were enforced everywhere. From the early meetings, they asked for volunteers for National Service – to enter the Home Guard, the Army, Navy and Air Force. The women, too, played a big part; the Women's Voluntary Service being an inspiration to everyone.
>
> Dr Gibbin was alert to every military change taking place. He knew that Major Protheroe-Beynon trained the men, and, when the regular morale-boosting marches took place around the town, he also took the salute. Dr Gibbin would have attended these occasions, and so would the entire town's population as our proud platoons marched with brass bands playing, and trombones and tubas.
>
> Most of the wartime work centred around the Memorial Hall, which became the military headquarters in the town. Dr Gibbin, over the road in Dolycwrt, would have heard and seen all the activity. Of course, the war changed his life considerably. He had always been an important person but, overnight, he became another man of extreme influence.

Dr Gibbin's first-aid expertise was now more vital than ever, as first-aid officers and units prepared themselves for serious work.

Examining the men enlisting, and attending to the wounded when they returned – as well as supporting the patients' families – demanded a lot of Dr Gibbin's time. We must not forget that many of the local doctors had been called away to duty early-on, leaving those at home with a considerable burden to carry.

During the early years of the war Haydn Lewis was a pupil at Whitland County School to which he cycled each day from Llanboidy carrying his gas mask. There would be training for the wearing of gas masks and Haydn remembers gathering in the old school corridors with other children for the air raid drills. Haydn recalls:

Things changed virtually all at once: no more street lights, enforced blackout and shutters to cover the windows. This was a nuisance for everybody, and it did not make life easy for Dr Gibbin and Dr Evans. Headlights had to be screened to dim the light. It was a strain to drive, because no one could see all that far. Speed had to be controlled; certainly no one could go fast.

In all this darkness, it was to be expected that accidents would happen. Perhaps people would collide with a bicycle, or fall in a ditch, and these problems added to the doctors' work. If Dr Gibbin was performing treatment in the surgery, he would have needed a light inside – probably a strong light, too – but this was not to be seen from outside. People used shutters and black curtains then. Or else they would hear a sharp reminder from the wardens to 'Put that light out!'. And Dr Gibbin had rather a lot of windows to cover at Dolycwrt.

I can remember breaking my arm during the war period, when practicing the high-jump, in Llanboidy. The County School sports day was approaching, and I landed awkwardly. So I crossed the field to Killa Jones, the carpenter, who was himself doing a bit of First Aid at the time. I needed a splint, so he planed a piece of wood. Then, when he started to bandage my arm, his housekeeper held open the pages of his book, while he followed the instructions as he went along.

I then went to see Dr Hugh Philipps at Clyngwynne, who referred me to the hospital in Carmarthen. When I returned to Dr Hugh Philipps in his little surgery in Llanboidy, some weeks later, to remove my dressing, his instruments would not cut the plaster. In the end he had to find some other way of finishing the job.

During these early days of the war, the late Mr William Gibbon opened the front of his house at Pwllywhead to the family of the late Dr Owen's sister, Mildred. Their home town Pembroke was under severe threat, because the fuel storage tanks at Pembroke Dock were being bombed. At their new farm residence, Mildred, her husband Thomas Harold Morris, and their children David, Jo and Kay, enjoyed the safe environment in Whitland's peaceful countryside.

Down the road in the County School, Maurice Dunbar, today of Snowdrop Cottage, can recall the days. Maurice, then a second year pupil, also remembers the Erith County School party arriving from Kent:

> Dr Gibbin took on a lot of patients all at once when the school children arrived. The teachers came with them and they usually had their lessons in the school, although sometimes Tabernacle vestry was also used. Erith was a boy's school, and, as youngsters, we built up good

friendships. Greenwich Junior School children were also welcome visitors. They were given lessons in the vestry of Bethania Chapel and were housed mainly in Velfrey Road. People who had a spare bedroom provided lodgings – called 'billeting' then.

Times were so different: very strict. If anyone had the cane in school, there would be a row at home from the parents. We knew right from wrong. The local policemen were very active, too. Although they were friends to everyone, they took no messing, and most people behaved. We would often see Dr Gibbin around the town and Dr Gibbin was a big man in our house. If you wanted to get better you listened to him. And he was an advocate of the coal fire – particularly for chest infections. In those days there were fires everywhere, including Dolycwrt.

I can remember Dr Evans arriving in Whitland. He was living in Gwyn Villa just across the road from Dolycwrt. He was a big sportsman, but rugby and football had virtually ended because of the war. Most of our men were in the battles. Dr Evans was a military man himself, and he was a strong presence in the town.

At the time, home-grown produce was important. With few jobs going, men and women helped on the farms. The more help the better, because the country needed food. I spent a school holiday at East Regwm farm. We had a lot of fun haymaking, and there was home-brewed beer for those who wanted it. But it was strong – you had to watch that.

Milk was provided in school as a healthy drink. Around the town, we used to see the farmers making their own horse and cart deliveries, and it was sold from jugs in half pint measures. No doubt, the doctors and nurses approved of this.

Dolycwrt misses Prime Minister
Winston Churchill's Visit

D URING THE MONTHS of August and early September 1940, patients visiting Dolycwrt would return home to their radio stations and learn of the bravery of the Royal Air Force fighter-pilots, who gallantly fought off the challenge of Germany's invading aircraft. News coverage of the Blitz came next, an exercise that Whitland could not escape, because planes were flying overhead towards the fuel tanks in Pembroke. Fifty miles away in the distance, Swansea would also be seen under attack as the eerie dark nights exploded into flashes of fire and light. Such activity continued until the following May, but despite feeling the weight of heavy bombardment and cruel destruction, Mr Churchill's Britain was winning these immensely important early battles of the war.

It is due to the incredible work of the medical and emergency teams that so many people were rescued from the upheaval of the bombings. Hospitals in the ravaged cities, and all around, were stretched to breaking point during extraordinary times when, following the night-time raids, people emerged from air raid shelters to be without homes and possessions in the morning. Doctors worked around the clock, and rescue operations never ended.

Dr Gibbin knew that hospitals such as those at Llanelli, Swansea, Neath, Port Talbot, Cardiff, would be bursting to breaking point during these air raids. This is why so many medical men were called to help neighbouring practices;

often leaving others to attend to their patients. Indeed, it was a case of everybody doing what they could. The Blitz saw the medical fraternity tested to the extreme, and it was no different at Dolycwrt.

In the cities, mounds of rubble lay all around. In the middle of it, was our inspirational leader, dressed in solemn black, with overcoat, homburg hat and cigar. Against a background of such destruction, he cut a forlorn figure, yet he was the nation's backbone now. And behind his saddened eyes, there was plenty more of his own fire as he planned a way forward to victory. But as springtime in 1941 burst onto the scene of British gardens and meadows, it was time for Mr Churchill to rally the troops in the provinces. This was to be a healthy change for our indomitable Prime Minister who went around raising people's spirits with his own special medical tonic.

With terrific secrecy and the strictest of schedules, Mr Churchill, accompanied by his wife, Clementine, and others, was making an Easter tour. From London, they travelled deep into the heart of west Wales – where, amazingly, both Dolycwrt and Whitland were to feature in a packed itinerary. The special train was, no doubt, gleaming as it went on its way; and accompanying this great man, as always, was his private secretary, John Colville whose memoirs[50] reflect upon these few days at the height of the war. The following are brief extracts:

Wednesday April 9th 1941
I listened to the Prime Minister's speech on the war situation in the House of Commons.

---

50 *The Fringes of Power: Downing Street Diaries 1940–1955, Vol 1,* John Colville, Sceptre Publishing.

Thursday April 10th
Left for a tour of the South-West with the Prime Minister
. . . We all slept on the train.

Friday April 11th
Good Friday. Reached Swansea at 8.00 a.m. and spent the
morning among the City's battered ruins. . .We went on by
train to Cardigan and motored from there to Aberporth on
Cardigan Bay . . . We slept on the train at a wayside station
called Whitland.

Saturday April 12th
Arrived early at Bristol. Breakfasted with the Prime
Minister . . . at the Grand Hotel.

There are people in Whitland today who remember Mr
Churchill's arrival on that Easter Friday. He was, in fact,
visiting the Aberporth Military Establishment to see a display
of rockets and weaponry. Of course, to get to Cardigan by
train meant a ride on the Cardi Bach line, starting out from
Whitland station, two hundred yards away from Dolycwrt.
In the Taf valley section, he would travel through Llanfallteg,
Login, Llanglydwen, Rhydowen, Llanfyrnach, Glogue and
Crymych, passing many of Dr Gibbin's country surgeries on
the way.

In Whitland it is a well known fact that during the war,
Mr Churchill had a bath in Llwynbedw, North Road, the
home of Alderman W. H. Mathias and his wife. Local people
remember seeing him walk through the entrance and up the
short driveway to the big Edwardian house. In those days,
North Road was so different. There were open fields where
the 'new' school buildings stand, and there was no Lôn
Hywel. In fact, there were very few patients' houses for the
doctors to visit beyond Llwynbedw; only hedges, grass and

trees. During this particular visit, strong looking men of stature – strangers, yet perfectly polite and pleasant – were seen around the town. These were Mr Churchill's security men guarding the country's biggest asset.

Les Rowlands, a local railwayman who dedicated so much of his life to the Cardi Bach line – the only route by rail to Cardigan – remembers the day as a young boy. During that Easter period in 1941, word had got around that something special was happening in town, and a crowd of people had gathered around the Station Square. It was at this very place that Dr Rowley Thomas is said to have met the great man, whose wife, Clementine, is reported to have taken Rowley by the arm. It was also here that Mr Churchill was seen both entering and leaving a big car. He was greeted with a warm Whitland welcome. 'Good old Winnie,' the locals shouted, and he politely smiled and gestured in response. Les explained what happened next:

> I remember seeing Mr Churchill on Whitland Square. I was a youngster then. He was getting out of a car. He took his hat off. He went up on the Cardi Bach line, and his special train was pulled by two local engines – there was a reserve engine that day, in case one broke down. But the train was so slow, with so many crossing points, and the steep gradient. I believe that he got out at Crymych and climbed into a car.

The time of Mr Churchill's return to Whitland is not known, but, as stated in Mr Colville's, memoirs, 'We slept on the train at a wayside station called Whitland.'

The late Percy Thomas – another great railwayman, who over the years attended dinners and events with many of the Dolycwrt doctors – once told me, 'Winston Churchill bunkered over there during the night.' We were both stepping-off a train one winter's evening, and he was pointing towards the old line alongside the former Farmers Cooperative. Again, this was shrouded in secrecy, and by day break, Whitland's 'Good old Winnie' was on the way to Bristol's Grand Hotel for breakfast.

For one gentleman in Whitland, who, during this historic episode, was to be no stranger to Dolycwrt, the departure of Mr Churchill brought a huge sigh of relief. The most important duty in a lifetime of police work had been duly discharged. This was Sergeant Job Enoch KPM[51] who lived with his family in one of the two end-of-terrace police houses in North Road. Sergeant Enoch was entrusted with the responsibility of overseeing the local security arrangements, with the help of Mr Churchill's private detectives. This meant guarding the Prime Minister during his entire time in Whitland, day and night. Sadly, Sergeant Enoch has long departed, but his story has been safe with his daughter, Miss Joyce Enoch, throughout all these years. It is a unique tale, and Dolycwrt – never far from the action – was meant to take centre stage:

Father's one regret was that he didn't ask Mr Churchill for his autograph. Of course, it was not the done thing; when you are on official duty looking after the Prime Minister, you cannot ask for his autograph, can you?

It was getting late afternoon and Mr Churchill's arrival was announced with very little notice. My father knocked on the door of Dolycwrt, and Dr Gibbin's housekeeper answered. 'May I see Dr Gibbin, please?' he asked. 'He'll be back before long,' she replied.

My father was not able to tell the lady that Mr Churchill intended visiting Dolycwrt that afternoon, and neither

---

51 King's Police Medal

was she going to reveal Dr Gibbin's whereabouts. But he returned to the surgery a few more times, without luck. Dr Gibbin, a bachelor then, was certainly away for the afternoon. His surgery-house was chosen because it was private, and near to the station. Of course, Dr Gibbin was also an important man.

Arrangements were then made for Alderman and Mrs Mathias to host the Prime Minister, at their home, Llwynbedw, North Road. Alderman Mathias was the power and the glory at the time, and had a big draper's shop in St John Street. Although Carmarthen was the county town, you bought locally in those days. Alderman Mathias took care of all the school uniforms for the Whitland County School. He also helped a lot of people to find jobs and was well respected and loved in the town.

At the time, I was only nine, and I certainly didn't know what was happening. But father made it clear that he was on important night duty, and that all the other policemen were also involved. Both Dr Gibbin and Dolycwrt missed the Prime Minister by a mere whisker. And, although this has been a well-kept secret over the years, I am now pleased to set the record straight.

There is one final piece of information to be shared concerning this memorable event in the history of both Whitland and Dolycwrt. There had been a belief in Whitland, and understandably so, that the Prime Minister may have taken his bath a few years later, when rehearsals for the D-Day landings brought him into Pembrokeshire. However, a visit to the premises by kind permission of its owner allowed me to see the complete picture. There at the top of the grand landing is the bathroom used by Mr Churchill. Inside is the old cast iron bath, high-sided and unaltered from that day.

On the back of the door is a notice, which has commemorated the event ever since:

The Right Honourable
Winston Spencer Churchill
when Prime Minister
took a bath here while on a tour
of military establishments
in Pembrokeshire
1941.

Of course, he had not been knighted then: his great legacy to the country and to the world being no more than work in progress at the time. It would all be so different after the war was won. On that Good Friday, April 11th 1941, he touched Whitland with his presence. For the people of the town, it was a proud day. And for Dr Gibbin and Dolycwrt, it was so nearly 'their finest hour'.

Mrs Emily 'Creswick' Williams is buried in Borth

M EANWHILE, FAR AWAY from Dolycwrt, Mrs Creswick Williams had been enjoying her retirement in Borth. Many years had passed since the death of her husband in 1916, but she had kept in contact with the Whitland area. On occasions she had stayed with Dr Bowen-Jones' widow and daughter, Caroline, at Glan-yr-Afon. It was there in the narrow lanes of Lower Village that these two ladies enjoyed setting out on their bicycles, usually for the nearby village of Meidrim a few miles away. Likewise on several occasions, Caroline and her mother visited Borth to stay with Mrs Creswick Williams. Her residence, Cliff Haven, was a substantial house, where, from the front room windows the huge expanse of sea in one of its many changing moods could be seen.

To make those visits to the Cardiganshire coast, Caroline remembers her mother hiring 'the village car', this being the only car in Llanboidy around the late 1920s. The driver collected them, and motored through delightful scenery amongst very light traffic, across the mountains and down the coast to Cliff Haven: a proper door-to-door service. When they were ready to return, the driver took them home:

> My mother and I enjoyed visiting Borth, and being chauffeured in that grand old car was a wonderful treat for us both. Of course, we received a warm welcome from Emily and her housemaid when we arrived.

We spent our time sitting around the fire talking, or playing games, and sometimes we went outside for a walk along the beach. But, on one occasion, we visited a neighbour's house. He happened to be a doctor, too, and we had an enjoyable meal together.

Mrs Creswick Williams was popular in Borth, devoting her time to St Matthew's Church, where her husband was buried. She died just before Christmas, December 1942, and was reunited with the great doctor at this beautiful place of rest.

Flying the Medical Flag in a Garrison Town

A ROUND THE MIDPOINT of the war, Dr Gibbin lost the services of his close partner, Dr Gwynne Evans. He was called to duty overseas, soon attending to the wounded behind the enemy line. Dr Gibbin, in need of help in Dolycwrt, was fortunate to have the assistance of a local young man, who was setting out on a very successful career, that would involve travelling the world.

This was Dr John Hirwaun Thomas, a native of Llanfyrnach, who had been brought up in a cottage called Gwernant, situated alongside a small brook that eventually finds its way into the River Taf. When he was a child, Dr Thomas' mother, Martha, used her front room as a sweet shop. Its location on the bend of the road that leads to Glandŵr is a typical rural setting in Wales, with the remains of an old smithy just across the road. Of course, Dr Thomas was a fluent Welsh speaker. He had attended Hermon School, then Cardigan Grammar – before the National School of Medicine, Cardiff, and the proud medical establishments of London.

Dr Thomas could relate to the war situation, because his father, William, had sadly died in the Great War. Dr Thomas was a fit and handsome man, and he certainly looked too kind to be a boxer, but this was one of his great loves. He taught the youngsters, including the Erith School children. He showed them all the tricks in the old gymnasium of the County School, and they were quick learners, too. Erith School members would not forget their Whitland experience, and met up with Dr Thomas, sixty years later, when they returned to a re-union in the town. Dr Thomas' niece, Creselda Davies, of Clynderwen, and her husband, James, were present that night.

'Hirwaun was guest speaker,' said Creselda. 'When he stood up to welcome the party from Erith, he said, jokingly, 'I can remember treating one of your friends in the old surgery. He had an appendicitis. I have often wondered if he is still alive.' Then someone stood up in the back of the room,

'It was me,' came the voice.

'Well, I am glad you are still with us!' Hirwaun replied.

Following his days at Dolycwrt, Hirwaun went on to be a chest specialist, posted to hospitals in England, before working abroad in far-away places including Trinidad, and the Caribbean, where he helped to start a new hospital in St Lucia. But he never forgot his roots, and wrote about his experiences, mostly in Welsh.

James was a pupil at the County School in the days of the Erith children, but he has no recollection of Dr Thomas at that time:

Hirwaun used to tease me about that – especially as he was teaching the boys in the gym. But I know he was fond of Dolycwrt, and worked well with Dr Gibbin. Hirwaun recognised that Dr Gibbin was a distinguished medical man in west Wales, whose clinical work was well-respected. He learnt a lot from him. Both Hirwaun and Dr Gibbin were passionate countrymen, enjoying the country way of life and the Welsh language. Dr Gibbin liked to be chauffeured, and Hirwaun enjoyed driving Dr Gibbin's rather wonderful cars. Of course, Hirwaun knew his way around the practice. Living in Llanfyrnach had taught him all the short cuts, too.

The doctors were to see Whitland inundated with Army personnel as a period of sustained military exercises took place in West Wales. Thousands of soldiers travelled through the town to camps near the coast of Pembrokeshire – giving Whitland all the hall-marks of a garrison town. There were American soldiers among them, and one division was stationed alongside Whitland's old Black Bridge. There was also an ordnance depot in the town, near today's rugby club. The American soldiers had a mighty presence and they integrated well with the locals. However, during these times of heightened activity, when so many soldiers were passing through the town, there would be some interesting times – and not always without incident. John Llewellyn explained:

> It was around this time that we had a riot in Whitland. It was a night that no one will forget, and I can't imagine what Dr Gibbin thought about it in Dolycwrt. It didn't take a lot for there to be a problem, because there were soldiers filling the streets, as well as neighbouring camps stationed outside Whitland. When something small sparked a disagreement, major incidents followed.
>
> That night, there were soldiers in Jeeps parading through the streets firing guns into the air. It was very serious. With so many men involved, our policemen couldn't possibly handle these problems. Sergeant Jenkins and P.C. Jones were in charge, and, in the end, they had to call the Home Guard out.
>
> People in Whitland had never experienced anything like it. It is a blessing that no one was hurt. No doubt, Dr Gibbin was waiting on stand-by. Of course, the soldiers had their own medical services, but Dr Gibbin had everybody else to consider. I am sure he was relieved to see the morning come around.

John Dunford, an ex-serviceman, knew all about these military exercises, which were in preparation for the D-day landings in Normandy. Camps were set-up all around the Pembrokeshire coast, and there were even Belgian soldiers taking part. They would jump off light landing craft out at sea, storming onto beaches only a few miles beyond the limits of the Dolycwrt practice, such as at Amroth, Saundersfoot, and Wiseman's Bridge. John described Whitland at the time:

I was a messenger-boy, and I had my own bike with A.R.P. painted on it. But I left it outside the Memorial Hall one night and it disappeared. Sometimes, during bomb alerts, we slept in the Hall on the floor. Then the all-clear sounded, and we knew that enemy planes had disappeared. The siren was at the Milk Factory so the noise was loud at Dolycwrt. And when it stopped, Dr Gibbin and his colleagues were free to continue with their visits.

The war years taught us all about the value of food, and looking after ourselves. This was good news for Dr Gibbin. We were all restricted by rations, and it worked to our advantage, because we were healthier. At such a difficult time for the doctors – who had to get to patients and hospitals when the entire place was under traffic patrol – this did, at least, provide some relief.

We all used to grow our own crop of vegetables, and we were allowed to have one pig at the bottom of the garden. We would feed it with edible waste, which we sometimes boiled. We didn't have fridges, so we would kill the pig whenever there was an 'R' in the month: such as in October. This meat would last a long time, supplementing our rations.

People also kept a few chickens for eggs. If you could catch a rabbit, it would make a nice meal, too. Those helping on the farms might receive some potatoes or vegetables, or maybe apples or blackberries when the time came round. But we had to work for our food. No one was overweight in those days. I am sure the weighing scales in Dolycwrt didn't see much use during the war.

As the end of conflict in Europe approached, *The Welshman* of May 11th 1945, described a plane crash in Whitland:

> On Friday last, a plane appeared to be in difficulty while flying over Whitland, carrying a crew of two. The local National Fire Service with their fire engine were soon on the spot, and found the plane burning fiercely.

It had been an incredible war, and Whitland and its doctors had experienced some unforgettable scenes. During its duration, the National Fire Service, the Air Training Corps, and the Young Farmers Club, had all emerged in the course of duty. Medicine had also learnt so much: aeroplanes falling from the sky, bombs, explosions, injured soldiers, and civilian casualties had all combined to take medicine's progress further. Penicillin had been tried and tested, and it would be staying too, soon to play a big role in Dolycwrt and every other surgery. As the long-awaited war celebrations drew closer, Edmund Richards – whose father was treated by Dr Gibbin after falling from a hay barn – was busy delivering milk in the town:

> I used to pass Dolycwrt every day on my milk cart. I was living in Penygraig, just outside Whitland, and there were always guards near New Inn. I had to explain what I was doing and display my official permit. They were careful who they let through.
>
> Victory in Europe brought terrific celebrations. It was a big day. There wasn't much beer left in Whitland that

weekend. At home we had just bought cabbage plants, and we had to finish our work before the drinking. 'You're not going down town in the day,' father said to me. He had never seen a field of cabbages planted so quickly.

Everybody was singing, and dancing, and merry. If Dr Gibbin had been in Dolycwrt, he would have heard the noise at the Grosvenor. There were fireworks going off and parties. That night we celebrated in style.

A Patient's Reflections –
and a Doctors' Reunion

'OUR NANCY,' from Cwmfelin Boeth, mentioned earlier as being Dr Owen's last patient, remembers the celebrations, and many more war experiences. She was still living with her parents just outside Whitland at Brynteg, Lampeter Velfrey. Together they farmed the land with good old-fashioned practices:

We all breathed a huge sigh of relief when it ended; enough was enough. It was time for life to get back to normal again. We all celebrated in style. In Bryn Sion, we had our own services of thanksgiving – most churches and chapels did, but there was wild excitement down at the Grosvenor Square.

I have so many different memories. At Brynteg, we used to plant a whole field of potatoes to sell in the war. We had two horses and a plough. The potatoes were planted by hand; perhaps as many as twelve people were involved. We sold them to the Farmer's Co-operative, although some were kept for our own use, or chopped up for the cattle in the winter.

There was usually a team of us working on the hay. The old machines, with blades on one side, were pulled by two horses on our farm; as well as the hay tedder, which turned the hay for drying in the sun. Some farmers had tractors by now, but we still used the traditional ways. Of course, we had to be careful, farm accidents would forever be keeping our doctors on their toes. Dolycwrt was well known for treating its farming friends.

To be truthful, I wanted to be a nurse, but on the farm we were doing work of national importance. I had to stay. One day a small aeroplane came over our field. I told Mam and Dad it was in trouble. Occasionally, stray planes would come down over the farms. They were British servicemen – sad days. The Women's Land Army was doing wonderful work across the country. They seemed able to cope with the hard work, all kitted out in their dungarees.

In the earliest period of the war, I was not well for a time, and I remember Dr Gibbin coming to see me with Nurse Sutton. I was rushed to hospital at Haverfordwest, because I was very poorly. Petrol was scarce because of the bombs falling on our fuel stores. One day, Dr Gibbin arrived by bicycle. Later he called with Mam and Dad. In the dairy we had hams hanging from the beams. Mam would give him some. He had worked hard for me; he had come back with good news. Sometimes, we would offer buttermilk, too. We always kept some milk to skim for butter. At that time, doctors were not paid from the country's budget as they are today. Often, instead of charging, they would accept a ham, or some butter. Things were different then.

I will never forget being a patient at the old County Hospital, Haverfordwest. They were dropping bombs on Pembroke Dock and the building would shake; and the sky would light up. The thud was so loud; it was very near from there. Everyone was frightened to death with those bombs. But the hospital staff carried on with their medical duties. They were courageous throughout, reassuring us at all times.

It was all so different when war ended and the church bells started to ring again. Thanksgiving services and parties for returning soldiers dominated the social scene, as a sense of togetherness prevailed around the town. The rations continued for some time, and, with little petrol available, people could not venture far away. For this reason, messenger girls and boys were seen everywhere making deliveries. They had a big basket in the front, and were often seen heading into the country. And, amongst the provisions they carried, there were often medicines from Dolycwrt Surgery.

For Dr Gibbin more work lay in store because the local athletes were thirsting for a game of rugby. It had been a long wait. Flying down the wing for Whitland Rugby Club's post-war team was Maurice Dunbar, soon to join the Royal Artillery himself. Danny Stephens was the secretary, and the teams changed in the Fisher's stables. This was a long single-storey building in front of the Fishers Arms, but it has gone now. Maurice remembers turning right through an old gateway before the school. There was usually a nice crowd waiting in the park, including qualified first-aid men, because these matches could be quite bruising encounters.

Rugby was a good social game then. It was well supported by the family. But we used to get into some real scuffles with the local teams. There were craftsmen at that. You had regular customers. They would look around, see the referee heading in another direction, and Bang! Games were physical. Besides Pembrokeshire matches, we played teams like Penclawdd, Llandybïe and Ammanford. We would meet up with colliers and farmers. They were hard men.

The town was full of qualified first aid men in those days. They had passed exams and knew exactly what to do. But

Dolycwrt was just across the road if things got serious. We knew we'd be looked after there.

It was around this time that Dr Gwynne Evans was returning from his military duties abroad to be reunited with Dr Gibbin. Coming from Burry Port, near Llanelli, it is hardly surprising that he was a keen rugby enthusiast, fully aware that a successful club gave the town a big lift. He added his weight to the cause, enjoying a close rapport with the players, and making sure that they were strong and healthy to get onto the rugby field. Affectionately known as Dr Bach ('bach' being a term of endearment in the Welsh language), he shared an interest in most things.

Dr Evans and Dr Gibbin would, by now, be noticing the Memorial Hall opening its doors for film shows. Initially booked for Wednesday evenings – before Thursdays became the preferred day for viewings – this was the start of cinema activity in the town, as noted in the Hall committee's minute book, on Tuesday, June 18th 1946:

> Application received from Sound Services Limited, London and the Cinematograph Presentations Guild, London, for the hire of the hall for the purpose of showing 'talking films.'

Both of the Dolycwrt doctors had a genuine interest in another extremely popular pastime in Whitland. Horse racing – staged in the wide-open fields of Rhosgoch farm, Cyffig – brought hours of local competitive sport, and was supported by large crowds from far and wide. Already, similar events were taking place at St Clears and Llanglydwen and, as neighbouring villages like Llanboidy had in earlier days enjoyed equestrian events, the Whitland races drew on established local crowds.

Arriving along the packed narrow lanes between Cyffig and Tavernspite was, itself, a spectacle but the fun was backing a horse and seeing it sprinting for the finishing post. There was a local flavour, too: the Yelverton Stakes and the Trevaughan Handicap were just two of the races, of varying lengths. Of course, accidents and mishaps could be serious. Jockeys were known to have heavy falls, so there was always a strong representation from Dolycwrt. Doctors Gibbin and Evans did not need a lot of persuasion. They were two real enthusiasts, taking their medical bags along just in case.

With the arrival of 1947 came a long period of freezing cold weather and snow. The ground was rock hard to quite a depth and, with little available fuel and obvious problems for the trains, the country was slowly grinding to a halt. Whitland was not spared the commotion, where drifting snow was seen rising to the height of the telegraph poles. For the doctors, it became almost impossible to get around, although Dr Evans had other ideas. Edmund Richards again explains:

> I remember the snow was on the ground, and my aunty was ill. She was living in a house that we had built on the farm. People were struggling to travel anywhere then. But Dr Evans got hold of an old cob at Penycoed. Then he came out to see my aunty on horseback. I remember meeting him at the top of the lane. 'Which way did the hounds go?' he asked me. He was a terrific character.

By now, Whitland had produced powerful boxers who had flown the town's flag for many years. Around this time, railwaymen like Frank Leggatt, Uri John and Owen Edwards were bringing honour to the locality with success in the national railway competitions. For this reason, Ron Taylor continued to bring his travelling boxing circuit to events in Whitland for quality bouts with the Whitland boys. Dr Evans was involved with this, not only attending to the men, but sometimes climbing into the ring himself and taking part. Clearly, he was no stranger to boxing from his military days, and it was a determined Dr Evans who ducked and dodged the punches, blood pouring from his nose, as youngsters at the ringside shouted their encouragement, 'Don't hit the Doctor.'

There is no doubt that Dr Evans enjoyed a close friendship with Dr Gibbin, supporting him up to the hilt as more patients joined Dolycwrt's expanding practice. Indeed, their partnership was strong and successful, steadying Dolycwrt's path during the crucial period leading up to, and beyond, the introduction of the National Health Service. In many respects, they shared similar attitudes and country interests, and it was during these years that they were both building new houses in the town. Dr Gibbin was moving to the east of Whitland, to Hafodwen, while Dr Evans was building Red Roofs (today's vicarage), in North Road. David Kuhl can remember the time:

> We often saw the two doctors around town together. At one time they both had Landrovers. Then they both built very fine houses. They were similar in many ways.
>
> I can remember Dr Gibbin calling at Dôl y Coed farm, when I was living and working there as a young man. He was very fond of the place and attended to the family's medical needs. We were milking a few cows in the old fashioned way, and we were also renting a small field nearby at New Inn. It was full of thoroughbred Rhode Island Red chickens in extended coops, and was quite a sight. Dr Gibbin was fascinated by what we were doing.
>
> Before building Hafodwen, he soaked the wood in the streams around Whitland. Dr Gibbin was exact about

these things; he knew what he was doing. I was one of the few people who worked on his driveway entrance. When the house was completed, it was considered an outstanding achievement; we were all proud of our contributions.

Dr Evans moved out of Gwyn Villa, opposite Dolycwrt, as soon as his house was completed in North Road. It was a large building, very private, in its own grounds, and everybody admired it. I can remember being with Dr Evans in some social gathering not long afterwards when a lady approached him,

'Dr Evans, you have the most beautiful house,' she said. 'I wouldn't mind owning that.'

'Neither would I,' was his quick response. 'Neither would I.'

The National Health Service

O N JULY 5th 1948, the National Health Service arrived, providing a range of free health care services. Simply, this meant that both adults and children would not have to pay for doctors, dentists, opticians, hospital treatment or medicines, while benefits for the unemployed, sick and elderly were also reviewed. This new system was the work of Welshman Aneurin Bevan, Minister of Health for the Labour Government. In return for providing such generous medical care, and having overcome stiff resistance to its implementation, Mr Bevan expected an improvement in the nation's health.

This was one of many changes taking place to build a better Britain following the ravages of war, as industries and services became part of a greater nationalisation programme. It is often said that war changes the course of history. Equally, it is clear that whilst our men and women fought together in both world wars, it is no coincidence that measures were being introduced to bridge gaps in sickness and welfare needs. The intentions of the National Insurance Act of 1911, introduced by David Lloyd George, and the report of Sir William Beveridge in 1942, both mirrored the purpose of the later National Health Service Act of 1946, which came into force two years later.

For the people of Whitland, and everyone across Britain, this was a huge changeover. Free dentures, glasses, medicines, and hospital treatment, was an amazing turn of fortune. It heralded the dawn of a new day. As for the doctors, there was initial uncertainty, mixed feelings and concern but, in the long run, it brought to an end the difficulties of obtaining payment from patients. This had been a problem especially when doctors charged per visit, and could not get an answer when they arrived on the doorstep of patients who were recovering. All this changed overnight.

Aneurin Bevan was born in Tredegar, a strong coal mining area. He was from a large family and followed his father into the mines, although it was as a trade union activist that Aneurin made his mark. No doubt the hardship that he witnessed in early life shaped his later political career, whereby he always did his utmost to support the hard working population. He demonstrated terrific passion for the National Health Service. Indeed, he resigned a few years later when certain benefits were withdrawn.

During those summer months in 1948 volumes of administrative changes took place. The State stepped in to assume overall control, and Regional Health Boards were set up to administer events. Of course, the very many municipal and voluntary establishments all over the country – including the two local hospitals that had served Dolycwrt so well, the Priory Street Hospital at Carmarthen, and the County Hospital at Haverfordwest – were all affected. This meant that after decades of control, the existing management committee's functions came to an abrupt and sad end. Indeed, despite the best intentions of Aneurin Bevan, many had mixed feelings about the new system, and this was captured by W. L. Richards, in his book *The County Hospital Story*:

> Under the new set up, the hospital went on to an eminently successful phase in its career, although many thought something was lost by the end of the voluntary system.

Pembrokeshire was immensely proud of the highly successful hospital it had supported for so many years.

It is a huge coincidence that the arrival of the National
Health Service in 1948 coincided with the 50th anniversary
of Whitland's Surgery at the Dolycwrt premises. Since Dr
Creswick Williams took ownership in 1898, so much had
happened in both life and in medicine; and, through all
the days – rain or shine, war or peacetime – Dolycwrt had
retained a stately and dignified presence in a little town whose
fortunes had changed and would change again.

This same year, 1948, brought news of progress in heart
surgery. Now the pace of change was beginning to gather
speed, and the arrival of the N.H.S. would be a landmark –
indeed a launching pad – as surgery and medicine were pro-
pelled into a more modern era, with more modern attitudes.

The earlier days at Dolycwrt were very different times for
Dr Creswick Williams. Such men were driven, devoted and
determined, wrapped up in a love of medicine, when life was
harsh, resources were few, and transport was limited. While
they were well remunerated in their particular era, the act
of giving service seemed to provide the greatest reward. It
is with grateful thanks to *The Welshman* that their deeds
have already been recorded. And, there are so many more
examples: such as when, in 1891, Dr John Phillips was
urgently called to the railway station, where a young boy with
a crushed leg, needed an immediate amputation, and when,
in 1900, Dr Creswick Williams was summoned to the same
venue to attend to a distressed railway passenger, whom he
examined in the comforts of the Yelverton Hotel.

Dr Owen's kindnesses were many, and there are stories
about him helping a woman when delivering her third child,
before he had received payment for the first. Other instances

of his good nature were mentioned earlier by Caroline Rees-Davies, whose father, Dr Vaughan Bowen-Jones, was once called to attend to a woman with many children, who asked for medicine.

'But it is not medicine you need,' he said to her. 'You must have coal and wood for your fire, and food and clothes for your children.'

He then acquired provisions to help her on her way.

'Doctors in those days had grandeur,' Caroline told me. 'They were great people and had a different aura. When my father walked into the village everyone knew him as the doctor, someone of great importance and someone they were pleased to now. They had a way of treating patients kindly.'

Caroline also worked with Dr Gibbin for a short while. She helped him with his paperwork and accounts at Dolycwrt, sometimes working late into the evening. No doubt, he was assessing the sweeping changes of 1948 because, besides being a country doctor, he did specialised hospital work, too. Sometimes patients would call to see him at Dolycwrt and, upon examination, he would say,

'Now it will have to be the hospital for you. Leave it to me, and I will get you admitted.' Then, a week or so later they would report to see the hospital specialist in Haverfordwest, or wherever, and they would meet up again with Dr Gibbin.

'Dr Gibbin had two or even three cars,' Caroline explained, reflecting upon an amusing story from the past. 'They were nice, substantial cars, but for some strange reason, they were all out of action one day. In desperation, he turned to me,

"Carrie," he said, "would you mind driving me to a patient without delay? It is an important visit; I must get there."

He was a big, mighty fellow.

"If you can get into my little car, then I will gladly drive you," I replied.

I took him as fast as I could to the place where the patient was desperately ill. On the way back, I will always remember him turning to me and saying,

"Carrie, do you know . . . you put great fear into me earlier."

He could be very amusing and, no doubt, he was a very brilliant man.'

Dr Rowley Thomas – the Perfect Hero

Iₙ 1949, whitland people shared the sad story of another departure. One of the town's greatest men – and ambassadors – was laid to rest after an extraordinary life. He is a man who will not be forgotten in the countryside surrounding his beloved Henllan Amgoed, or in the urban setting of London Welsh Rugby Club, which he helped to found way back in 1885.[52] This is a man who was widely loved by most: known as Rowley, 'Dr Rowley,' 'Dr Parke' or, officially, as Dr Roland Lewis Thomas, of Parke farm.

If ever a man stood out as a leader, it was Rowley. He was a dedicated doctor, an excellent rugby player, a first class shot, and a superb cricketer. He played billiards, led the hunt, and loved fishing, animals, and all aspects of traditional country life. As an international rugby player, he threw his burly body at the best of the English, Scottish and Irish packs. Then in the Great War, he appeared on four of the fronts. Later he became a highly respected public figure, serving as both a councillor and coroner. Blessed with a sharp mind, and spontaneous wit, Rowley appeared as free as a bird, sometimes seen later in life running through the main streets of Whitland, pretending to pass a rugby ball. At heart he was peaceful and he could not hide his inner contentment and pride, because his mischievous smile gave the show away.

It is with thanks to both Natalie Winton and to Paul Beken, of London Welsh Rugby Club, that so much detail has

---

52 *Dragon in Exile*, Paul Beken, London Welsh Rugby Club.

been found about this popular doctor. 'I have quite a lot of information on Rowley Thomas,' wrote Paul to Natalie, 'He was indeed a founder member of the London Welsh Club, and a very significant one at that.' Paul provided extracts from his earlier work, *Dragon in Exile,* written in the 1980s to mark the Club's centenary, besides other information on Rowley.

Born in the early 1860s in Henllan Amgoed, he was educated as a schoolboy at Llandovery College. After becoming an LSA (Licentiate of the Worshipful Society of Apothecaries) in 1890, he returned to London in 1908 to acquire an LMSSA (Licentiate in Medicine and Surgery, Society of Apothecaries) before crossing the water to Ireland in 1909 to do a Diploma in Public Health, at the Royal Colleges of Physicians and Surgeons, of Ireland.[53] Rowley played 69 times for London Welsh between 1885 and 1892,[54] and hardly ever missed a match. In his book, Paul states:

> Rowley was a man of immense physique, one of the most dominating forwards of his time. He played for Wales between 1889 and 1892 and, apart from captaining London Welsh, he also played for Llanelli, Middlesex, and University College Hospital. He was a familiar figure in the players' enclosure at international matches for years after his playing days were over.

In the 1889–90 season, Rowley took over the club captaincy; and, on a wet Thursday afternoon at Raynes Park, Llanelli were remembered as being the first team to travel from Wales to play against London Welsh. Again, in his work, Paul described the events:

53 The Royal College of Physicians of Ireland.
54 Notes provided by Mr Paul Beken.

The *Llanelli Guardian* correspondent recalled that the Scarlets, on the last leg of an English tour, were met at Paddington 'by a jolly crew of London Welshmen, including Mr R. L. Thomas, who made the arches of the monster station echo with their enthusiastic cheers. We were now piloted to the Prince of Wales Hotel. Here a splendid supper was already laid hot and steaming for us, and all set to in thorough good earnest.

Llanelli narrowly won the game. Afterwards London Welsh invited their opponents to 'a splendid spread at the Horse Shoe, Tottenham Court Road . . . never do I remember a more jovial, more hearty, more patriotic, more enthusiastic gathering.'

When serving in the Great War, he found time for a fishing expedition on the River Nile. Paul wrote of this escapade:

It was said that he hooked such an enormous fish that it took him a full hour to land it, and when he did so, the level of the river went down by four inches!

This is a story typical of Rowley's humour!

Rowley had his own practice at Parke farm, in the beautiful countryside of Henllan Amgoed. He was a friend of Dr Creswick Williams and Dr Owen, and they often teamed up for second opinions, and helped each other. He was narrowly beaten by both these doctors, on separate occasions, to the vacant Medical Officer's post, but neither could rival him on the cricket or sporting field. In local politics he was a force to be reckoned with and, in the early 1900s, he worked tirelessly for the beautiful stone bridge at Cwm Miles. He also supported Whitland Rugby Club, and became its President.

Indeed, Rowley enjoyed doing favours for everybody. David Kuhl, mentioned earlier, once had an accident when he took his horse to the blacksmith at Henllan Amgoed. This was just a short walk from Rowley's home farm, Parke:

> When the old mare was being shoed, a hot piece of metal flew through the air, catching me on my open wrist. It severed the vein and Rowley wasted no time in treating my wound, in his surgery. 'Now go to see your own doctor in the morning,' he said to me in his loud voice. The next day I walked into Dolycwrt. Dr Gibbin took a look at my wound, 'Who did this for you?' So, I told him. 'You should have come straight to me.' They were good friends, but also keen rivals.

Rowley is buried in the old Henllan Amgoed Church alongside the green rolling hills, miles away from the famous fields of Old Deer Park, in London, where he raced around taking the knocks, before getting up and taking some more. Likewise, in the Great War, Rowley was no different. After being injured and carried from the field, he recovered and returned to duty.

Whilst recuperating, a garden fete was held at his home, Parke. This was in 1916, to help the Red Cross fund. In *The Welshman* of August 18th that year, it was reported that a large crowd gathered for tea and games, including tennis. There were stalls selling various items and, later in the day, the Whitland Male Voice Choir entertained everyone. But soon after this, Rowley was on his way again, returning to active service in Egypt, and other war fronts. He could be strong, but he could be gentle, too. And he was always the perfect hero.

Buried with his hunting gear, Rowley's funeral service ended with the sound of the huntsman's horn. Amongst a big crowd of mourners in the winter scene of that January day were his friends from Dolycwrt . . . Doctors Gibbin and Evans. They would miss Rowley, too, and had come to say their last farewell.

Patients 'Rock Around the Clock' – as Dr Roland Lewis Arrives

Medicine and surgery had made quite a journey from the days of the priest-physicians, and had now entered the era of kidney transplants. Clearly, the period following the National Health Service was defining a different era in medicine but this was also true of other aspects of life. Whitland, for instance, had now been blessed with a modern sewage system. The old doctors would take delight in knowing that the days when the faithful horses dragged the old cart up and down the back lanes in the dead of night, were long gone. This was to happen no more. The large metal drum that sat in the cart had been taken into the countryside, and emptied, for the last time as progress, everywhere, continued onwards and upwards towards pastures new and green.

In 1953, both Whitland and Dolycwrt experienced the excitement of the Queen's Coronation. As a memorable golden carriage was drawn along London's Mall, flags and bunting adorned Whitland's town centre buildings. Meanwhile, people were now gathering around new television sets happily watching the ceremony unfold. As ever, the Log Book of the Council School recorded the local events that day:

> Today, Tuesday, Her Majesty Queen Elizabeth II was crowned. The event was suitably celebrated in Whitland – the houses and streets were gaily decorated with flags and bunting. In the afternoon, the junior boys and girls

gave a dancing display at the Grammar School. Sports for children were held on the Grammar School field and tea for all was provided at the Grammar School dining hall. The celebrations ended with a fireworks display in the park.

By now, all cinema activity had been moved from the Memorial Hall in Whitland, just a short walk away to the Town Hall in King Edward Street. It is there that a well known local businessman, Mr W. S. Cole, ran regular shows, the venue being known as the 'Coleseum' [sic]. In providing Whitland with more frequent films he greatly added to the town's entertainment, and many of Dolycwrt's patients remember the days.

Roy Harverson was born during the war years when Dr Hirwaun Thomas served at Dolycwrt Surgery. Then a young boy, he loved to attend the film shows. He remembers some of the earlier productions, which included *The Everest Expedition*, *The Dancing Years*, and *The Queen's Coronation*. He said that the 'Coleseum' was open six nights of the week, and the film programme changed every Wednesday. In the darkness of the show, some of the boys would quietly move from the cheaper shilling seats to the bob and six penny seats, if they were empty, and Roy was one of these. He is also the first to admit that he was often caught and sent back.

One of Roy's favourite memories involve the showing of *Rock Around the Clock*. This was in the medical era when Nurse Evans, from Penycwm, was respected throughout the area as a district nurse; when health visitors were making regular visits to the schools, when Nurse Nan Davies was becoming well-known for carrying-out health inspections, and when the Memorial Hall was available for clinics. Cinema nights were appealing social occasions, professionally run, with usherettes, projectionists, local commercials at the interval, and a popular next-door attraction, the Dorothy Café. Roy can remember an extraordinary buzz during the showing of Bill Haley's great work. There was electricity in the Coleseum, as Dolycwrt patients, young and old, nodded their heads back and fore, as they shifted around on their seats. Roy continues:

I used to go to the surgery often. There was a little dispensary in the waiting room, where there would be room for about six people to sit, while the rest waited outside. Doctors Gibbin and Evans were the main men, but we were starting to see other doctors helping out as locums.

As pupils of the primary school, we often used to have an appointment with the visiting Health Inspector. This was held in the school boardroom, the room on the right under the bell tower. I remember our parents were invited on one occasion and my mother was quite upset about my medical report that day. She went straight across the road to have a word with Dr Gibbin. Minutes later Dr Gibbin came over the school. He knew my health records intimately, and he had a few words to say to the inspector that day.

Dr Evans used to visit my elderly granny. She thought the world of 'Dr Evans,' who made a habit of calling on her on his way home from Llanboidy. When he was unable to help her medically, he would still call socially, sometimes with home-brewed beer. Of course, his visits were a real tonic for my granny in more ways than one.

Roy shared one more of his favourite childhood stories:

As a boy, I used to look forward to having my hair cut with Wynford Harries in the middle of St John Street. For me, having a haircut took longer than usual. I remember going into Wynford's shop and seeing a few wooden chairs to sit on – a little bit like a doctor's waiting room – while we waited our turn. There was a cabinet in the corner, with a few bottles of lotion, and one or two pots of Brylcreem. Because I was small, Wynford put a piece of wood across the solid arms of a wooden chair for me to sit on – always positioned near to the window – and he wrapped a sheet around my neck. Then he would start with his clippers.

His mother lived in the back and she would bring him a cup of tea. But Wynford, a well-loved character in Whitland, was known to prefer something stronger. When he put down his cup on the mantelpiece, I knew this would be a long job. 'If Mam comes in, tell her I am making a phone call,' he would say. Then he would head straight across the road to the Railway Tavern (today it is the Taf Hotel), where he would keep an eye on the shop from the window.

John Davies is another with similar memories of Wynford's hair-cutting days. John, mentioned earlier because he grew up in Dr Gibbin's neighbourhood, remembers the local characters at that time, most of whom were patients at Dolycwrt. He used to visit an elderly couple, who were both a little deaf, and remembers the lady pouring tea into her husband's cup from the old teapot. As it filled quickly to the brim, her husband would call out,

'Stop! Stop!'

'Don't be crude Dan,' she would reply. 'You should shout, "Halt, Halt." We have visitors.'

And, as regards the Whitland barbers, John had his own story to tell, which involved Dr Gibbin:

After Wynford's day, Fred Thomas had a barber's shop in King Edward Street. Time had moved on a little by now, and Fred had bought himself a swivel-chair. I remember being there on a very wet morning when, perhaps as many as eight people were in the queue. I was waiting my turn, too. That day Fred was using a new invention, the electric clippers, and this was for the very first time. Standing in the doorway observing this breakthrough was Dr Gibbin.

Now in those days it was usual for a doctor to jump the queue, because they were important, they were not usually kept waiting. But that morning Dr Gibbin made it clear that he was happy to wait. He was intrigued by what was happening; he wanted to see for his own eyes that there were no bad effects coming from this new device. I remember this clearly. He was a terrific character, and I knew him well. But he was also a thinking man; this was Dr Gibbin playing safe.

In the mid 1950s, Dr Gibbin and Dr Evans secured the help of a popular local doctor who had earlier attended Whitland Grammar School, where he enjoyed the school rugby and sports scene as well as his studies. Dr Roland J. Lewis qualified in 1952 and spent two years in Dolycwrt between 1954 and 1956. Marian his widow recalls the days:

> It was a long time ago, and I remember Whitland being so busy in those days. Besides the railways and the milk factory and a growing grammar school, Whitland had a good shopping centre. There were so many nice shops. I remember W. H. Mathias, and Monty Davies and a dressmaker's shop called Rosser and Bowen. I was fond of that little dress shop, where you could buy smart clothing and accessories, like scarves and gloves and bags. It was genteel. You could find most things in Whitland then. Roland was very busy in Dolycwrt. He enjoyed getting out into the countryside on visits, and he took his turn running the smaller surgeries at Llanglydwen and Hermon and in those other pretty little villages.

With so much happening in Whitland, Roland had the chance to set up on his own, and he worked at Norton House in King Edward Street for nearly ten years. We were living at Trefethin, North Road, and Whitland was a friendly place, where Roland got involved in community life. During the war he had served in India with the 5th Regiment of the Royal Gurkhas so he became an active member of the local British Legion branch for many years. There was always a strong medical presence in their meetings, because so many of the doctors had served in the war, or attended National Service abroad. Dr Hugh Lewis-Philipps was president for years, and there was Dr Gwynne Evans and, of course, Dr Penn later became involved.

At the time when Roland practised alone, it was difficult to find a locum, so his hours were long. When he was asked to join Dr Peter Williams' Group Practice in Narberth, this seemed to be the right move for us, and we quickly settled there. But it was sad leaving Whitland. We left with fond memories.

Roland also used to work at the Medical Hall chemist shop. He was there with Eddie Evans, my Uncle Ed. After schooling, Roland qualified as both a pharmacist and optician, before he entered medical school at St Mary's Hospital in London as a mature student. It was at Medical Hall, that I met Roland for the first time. That was when we were both young. College life and the war intervened before we met up again, much later in 1953. Then we married in the summer of 1954, during Roland's days at Dolycwrt.

Dr Penn visits Hafodwen for an Interview

As DR ROLAND LEWIS prepared to move from Dol-ycwrt, a young and ambitious doctor was enjoying every moment of his locum work in the beautiful Welsh countryside of Newcastle Emlyn. For five months Dr George Penn, my father, had been helping Dr Trevor Davies by running his practice since he had become unwell. He had only been reunited with his wife, Peggy, earlier in the year, after serving his National Service duties in Nigeria. Indeed, it is in this quaint little town that they had started married life, and this is where they wanted to stay. For Dr Penn the job was enjoyable and he liked the patients, who nearly all spoke Welsh. They were all so pleasant to him; and, although he was on call the whole time, he was rarely disturbed at night. The practice was almost entirely rural, and extended to the popular holiday venues on the coast, including Aberporth, Tresaith, and Llangrannog.

There is no doubt, whatsoever, that Dr and Mrs Penn saw their future in Newcastle Emlyn. They had immediately settled in this peaceful farming area, and equally they were at home in their small flat. However, Dr Davies had made good progress and wanted to take over the reins once more. This meant that Dr Penn was no longer needed. Having heard that Dr Gibbin, in Whitland, was looking for an assistant, he travelled to meet him. However, if Dr Penn had known that Dr Davies was then going to invite him back only three weeks later, things would have been different. Below is an extract of a dinner speech that Dr Penn made in the locality years later, describing his first meeting with Dr Gibbin:

> One day, Peggy and I made the lovely cross country trip from Newcastle Emlyn – via Boncath, Crymych, Efailwen and Login – to Whitland for an interview with the late Dr Phillip Gibbin, at his beautiful home, Hafodwen. Dr Gibbin seemed to be a large but benevolent gentleman, wearing plus fours – as was his wont – who had obvious and understandable pride in everything about him: his wife, family, home, profession, FRCS, and the whole practice area, which included the countryside of his native Login. He was very impressive, but very likeable too, and Peggy and I actually enjoyed that visit to Hafodwen very much. There we had the joy of hearing, before we left, that he had decided that I would be his assistant as from September 8th 1955, when I joined him, and Dr Gwynne Evans, at Dolycwrt Surgery.
>
> In those days, St Mary's Street was an extremely busy and, perhaps, noisy street, where men and women in the employment of the Dairies recycled the milk churns off the lorries and onto the platform. Apart from this landing bay, and a small entrance into the Dairies, this particular side of St Mary's Street was built up with houses and shops over the entire length. Soon after coming to Whitland, there was a night call on rather a cold night to Tavernspite and I accompanied and drove Dr Gibbin. When we arrived back at Hafodwen, he insisted that I go inside for a while, and my welcome at that time of night – three o'clock – was amazing. I was given a whiskey. 'It was a cold night', he explained to Mrs Gibbin; then Mrs Gibbin presented us both with a very generous ration of bacon and eggs, which we unhurriedly enjoyed in the early hours, and there we

chatted 'tally ho'. But then he asked me, what was to be, a vital question, 'What do you think of Whitland?' . . . to which I replied, 'Not very much'.

In fairness to myself, I had not been in Whitland long enough to know anything about it; but Dr Gibbin took it upon himself to extol its virtues in a big way. He told me much of the history: Hywel Dda, the famous Whitland Abbey, the local *cromlech*, the coming of the railways and the growth of the milk factory. He mentioned the schools, the primary, the grammar and the secondary modern, and he told me about the successful rugby and cricket teams. Then he explained about the park; the late Dr Owen and Dr Rowley Thomas; the public houses; the Whitland choir; the church and chapels, as well as the Cardi Bach railway, which had often carried him to Whitland as a boy. And he won me over, and I think he planted in me a liking and pride for Whitland, which has remained with me ever since.

Born in Cardiff, but with an early upbringing in Bryn-menyn, near Bridgend, Dr Penn was educated at the Royal Masonic School for Boys, Bushey, in Hertfordshire. This was an outstanding establishment, traditional, strict and challenging, with excellent running tracks, sports fields and general classroom facilities. After settling there, his studies were interrupted at a young age when he became ill. In the peacefulness of his hospital wards over many weeks, he appreciated the kind attention bestowed upon him by the nurses and doctors. By the time he had recovered his health, he had already made the first big decision of his life: he wanted to become a doctor.

From that moment on, he laboured hard at his studies with every possible endeavour. To a great extent, he was encouraged by his family. His mother was the widow of a Merchant Navy sea captain. She drove him hard, and so did her sisters; she was one of six daughters, most of whom were teachers. They cajoled and challenged him, and gave great encouragement, too. Dr Penn's Auntie Mattie was the headmistress of Colwinston Junior School, near Cowbridge, where pupils excelled themselves under her. For Whitland's doctor there were great expectations and, of course, he delivered.

At the time of his studies at the National School of Medicine in Cardiff, he was living nearby at the Wyndham Hotel, Cowbridge Road, just a short walk from Ninian Park, the home of Cardiff City Football Club. His mother ran the enterprise, and, in fairness, she had occasion to handle some tough characters, and she did well. When, sometimes, she was beaten, she would play her last card:

'If you don't getttt owtttttt,' she would blast, 'then I will call my son!'

Upstairs, in his little study on the top floor, he would be busy drawing the aortic valves of the heart in the finest of detail. Of course, he would come down, and enter the frenzied excitement of the bar, but he was always too gentle to be awkward. And it was from these early days that he learnt the art of influencing, negotiating, tactfulness and diplomacy, which later served him well in all his serious campaigns.

After qualifying in 1951, Dr Penn reported to the small and delightful Llandough Hospital, a sea-front location where he assisted a Surgeon by the name of Mr Douglas Foster. Inspired by this gentleman, he took every opportunity to operate under his watchful eyes. Indeed he often referred to those days with Mr Foster – stating at the end of his career, 'There in Llandough, Cardiff, the seeds were sown of a delight in minor surgery, which stayed with me throughout.'

He then moved on to Neath General Hospital to do six

months of midwifery and gynaecology. 'It was at Neath that I met Peggy, who was telephonist and receptionist. Her voice would be heard all day when she was announcing on the loud-speaking system when somebody was wanted. She sounded really nice, and we got married.'

Firstly, Dr Penn did another six month stint, this time as House Physician, which started at Neath, but continued at Port Talbot, where he was also the Casualty Officer:

> I heard that Port Talbot Hospital couldn't get anyone as House Physician, so I asked if I could be transferred there, which they were pleased about. It was a small hospital, but it was also lovely, I thought. There was an Indian Surgical Registrar in residence, and he was a fantastic doctor and surgeon. It was an exciting and stimulating experience being with him, and meeting with the Port Talbot G.Ps., with whom we worked closely.

Then came his Army call up with the Royal Army Medical Corps. After attending initial training, which included the usual 'square bashing,' the next big event was his marriage to Peggy at Maes-yr-Haf Church, Neath, which stands alongside the east bound platform of the town's railway station. This happy occasion took place on a fine day in the spring of 1953. Dr Penn, often known to be late, was on time for this important event. He was there standing alongside Colin Evans, Best Man, at the front of the church as his bride, looking slim and resplendent in her beautiful pale blue patterned dress with matching hat, walked down the aisle with her brother, Gwyn, and her twin sister and bridesmaid, Glenys. After a wedding reception in the next street at Neath's Castle Hotel – famous for staging the meeting that led to the birth of the Welsh Rugby Union – the happy young couple left for Llanarth, near New Quay, Cardiganshire for their honeymoon.

It was only a few months later that Dr Penn received the news that he had an overseas post. It was to Nigeria, West Africa, for eighteen months. Now, he had to leave Peggy behind to join his regiment:

We left Blackbush Airport, somewhere near London, in a four-engine aircraft, called a Hermes, around mid morning in early June 1953 on the first stage of the journey to Algiers, North Africa. But after a few hours we could see that one of the propellers on the starboard side of the plane was absolutely still. It was decided that we return to Blackbush for engine repairs; so immediately we had another night in the U.K.!

The next day we got to Algiers and were put up in a nice hotel. And the day after, we continued southwards, flying over the Sahara Desert for several hours, before landing somewhere for refuelling. I remember stepping out of the aircraft into, what felt like, an oven; it was so very, very hot.

After arriving in Kano in the north of Nigeria, we flew down to Lagos on the coast, and there we were put up in a Military Hospital for a couple of weeks. The climate was warm, wet and humid and everyone perspired profusely. We accompanied the doctors of the military hospital in their work, and gradually became familiar with the medical problems and treatments of West Africa.

The main illness we ourselves had to guard against was Malaria. This was brought to people by the mosquito taking a bite, usually in the hours of darkness, between 7 pm and 7 am. Before darkness we had to have a bath, and get into long trousers and a shirt with buttoned sleeves, and footwear like soft leather boots, which we tightened to stop mosquitoes from getting to our legs. Then mosquito nets covered us in bed at night.

I was soon onward bound on a West African Airways flight to Kaduna, somewhere in the centre of Nigeria, before being sent by train on a two day journey to Emugu, South Eastern Nigeria. There I spent the next 15 months as Regimental Medical Officer to the 2nd Battalion of the Nigerian Regiment. Some of the soldiers were allowed up to four wives, so I had rather a lot of women and children to see as well as the officers, sergeants and soldiers!

The Africans were delightful people, and their children were adorable. They were always teasing one another and teasing me, and they were just bursting with rhythm; in fact, I once joined them at their local open air cinema, and, during the main film, the projector failed and the film stopped. In Britain, this would have started off a lot of moans, but not so in Emugu. All the Africans started to make rhythmical movements, until the whole place became almost a frenzy of beating drums, rhythm and swaying. The film was back running for about five minutes before everyone settled down to see it again.

After being in West Africa for 18 months, I was flown back home in time for Christmas 1954 and was reunited with Peggy. Then Peggy joined me in Aldershot for my last two and a half months in the Army.

Doctors Gibbin and Penn –
Two Doctors Full of Work

D R PENN HAD the greatest respect for Dr Gibbin, his senior colleague. When either of the two doctors was away from Dolycwrt on holiday, they communicated regularly by letter or postcard. Of course, there were no mobile phones then and when Dr Gibbin was returning home, he would be very precise, 'I will see you on Saturday – 3pm'. Dr Gibbin was equally formal; the same postcards opened with the words 'Dear Dr Penn'. There is no doubt, however, that they soon became very close, enhanced by Dr Evans' departure from the scene in 1958 to take-up a Regional Health Board appointment outside the area:

> At this stage, I was made a partner to Dr Gibbin. We took on a marvellous chap, Dr David Bayton, but he didn't stay long. We then had Dr John Merrell – or 'Dickie' as I knew him at medical college. He was Welsh speaking and very, very conscientious. I think he worked almost too hard.

At the time, Sir Eric Howells, former Chairman of the Conservative Party for Wales, occasionally visited Dolycwrt Surgery as a patient. Sir Eric has not forgotten the warm atmosphere of the old building, with its small rooms and narrow doorways, and shared a story about each of the two doctors at this time:

One of my earliest memories of Dolycwrt dates back to the time of Dr Gibbin, many years ago. We all entered the surgery through the back door then, and I would sit with the other patients in the small waiting room.

'Next!' he would call out, and, when it was my turn, I would step into the consulting room, where Dr Gibbin would be sat at his desk. When I needed a medicine, he would look over his glasses at me.

'Have you got a bottle?' he would ask.'

'Yes,' would be my reply. We would all carry a bottle to the surgery; Dr Gibbin had trained us well. Then he would go into his little dispensing room, and he would come out with a mixture. Dare I say, it was never a nice mixture.

I can also remember Dr Penn around this time, these being his early years in Whitland. He called to see me one winter's day when I was unwell. It was snowing, but that did not deter him. Equally, he was totally relaxed when his car got stuck in our lane, seemingly having all the time in the world. I had a bout of tonsillitis. For the next week, he called every day, and kept in contact with me until I was well again.

The close bond between the two doctors continued. Both valued many of the traditions of country life in west Wales, and they shared a love of Dolycwrt and all it represented as an old fashioned surgery. Indeed, they were of the same ilk as Dr Finlay and Dr Cameron, as portrayed in the delightful television series *Dr Finlay's Casebook*. Of course, since his arrival way back in 1932, Dr Gibbin had built up the practice through his expertise and great influence. It now stretched a few miles further north, beyond the parish of Eglwys-Fair-a-Churig, in Llanglydwen, which defined the northern boundary during Dr Creswick Williams' day. Although the branch surgeries were very active, all roads continued to lead to Dolycwrt as the medical establishment of the area.

At home Dr Penn often talked about Dr Gibbin. As a family, we used to go swimming in Amroth, indeed we once had a week's holiday in Amroth Castle, and he told us that Dr Gibbin was so happy in the area that he didn't care about venturing far away. Dr Penn also once said of his partner:

> It was a rich experience being with Dr Gibbin. He was a real countryman and a real country doctor. He was full of work and never was he happier than when he saw me busy.

One local person who knew Dr Gibbin well is Gwynfor Reynolds, whose son, Alan, is no doubt better known, because he was one of Whitland's greatest rugby players, performing for Swansea with distinction and representing Wales on three occasions, during the more modern, well televised, days of sport. Gwynfor was one of a number of chauffeurs who helped Dr Gibbin when on calls. He explained how this started:

> It happened when I was doing farm work, and I had been kicked on the knee by a cow. I went to the Bont surgery, Llanglydwen and saw Dr Gibbin. I returned there and when my knee was better, he asked me if I could drive a Landrover; then he asked me to drive him the next day.
>
> He was a terrific character and he liked to stop in a lay-by between Clynderwen and Llandissilio to have an Oxo drink. One day I was slightly late for him, and he knew exactly where to find me, because I was having a quick drink in the pub. 'Is my driver there?' he asked in Welsh on the telephone. Of course I was never late again.
>
> I did some farming for him when he moved to Hafodwen, because he had a few fields and kept cattle. On an-

other occasion, I was asked to paint one of the consulting rooms ready for Mr Dormer, the dentist, who used to hold a clinic at Dolycwrt.

Dr Gibbin always had a nice story to tell, which sounded funnier in Welsh. He once told me that he went to a home confinement. The woman was upstairs in the bedroom and her husband was frantically wandering around asking if there was anything that he could do. 'No,' he said sharply, 'You've already done enough.' He was a great man.

Dr Gibbin and his junior partner would have been thrilled when the new and modern section of Glangwili Hospital was opened by the Queen Mother on May 25th 1959. With such wonderful facilities coming into the heart of West Wales, this was seen as a major step forward for medicine on the local scene. But around this time there was news that would equally have saddened them both, concerning the closure of Penygaer School. Of course, for Dr Gibbin, this is where it all started in the early 1900s, just a short walk from his home farm in Login. Glyndwr Phillips, a pupil of the school long after Dr Gibbin's day, has a funny story to tell:

> I can remember throwing stones down the bank with my friends – it was a steep bank with a house at the bottom – and we enjoyed watching them bouncing over the roof. They would land then in front of the house. One day, the tenant of the house came up with a big bucket-full of stones. He knew when to come. We were all in class at the time, about twelve or fifteen of us. Then we had a big row – and that was the end of that.

In the Carmarthenshire County Archives, the School Log Book describes how the final days brought to an end an era that lasted nearly eighty years. In explaining how the number of pupils had fallen, and the inevitability of the school closure, the head teacher described the final visits of the police constable and the district nurse. Then the entry for March 25th 1959 referred to an event that Dr Gibbin may well have attended – surely, as one of the most qualified pupils in the history of the school. Below is an extract:

> This afternoon, friends and parents attended a short serv-ice to bring this school to a close. Penygaer was opened on Monday 5th November 1883. Today sees its closure and the end of my service as its head teacher. Looking back over the past 37 years, I am conscious of many blessings received.

Then, thanking his staff, the education officers, visiting inspectors, local school managers, and parents of the pupils, the gentleman ended his speech on a touching note:

> As for the little school itself, I love every stone in it, and its memory will never fade. It remains for me to write but one final word – 'Finis.'
>
> W. Rhydderch Evans, Head teacher, March 25th 1959

Looking back to the school's beginning in 1883, this was soon after Dolycwrt was built. It was also the time when Dr Creswick Williams was a medical student. The common denominator linking this first great doctor, and Dr Owen and Dr Gibbin was the simple fact that they had all carried Dolycwrt's mantle into a new era. December announced the arrival of another Christmas Season but 1959 would be a time of immense sadness in Whitland and Login, and all over the Practice area. Like Dr Creswick Williams, and Dr Owen – and now Penygaer School – Dr Gibbin's days had also come to an end.

Dr Holding arrives in Dolycwrt
as the Cardi Bach Era ends

NEWS OF DR GIBBIN's sudden departure travelled
quickly around a community that shared an overwhelming sense of loss. The tributes flowed; the *Carmarthen
Journal* leading with the heading 'Esteemed Personality:
sudden death of Dr Gibbin, Whitland.' In an article paying
great respect to Dolycwrt's late doctor, it also highlighted Dr
Gibbin's commitment to his profession until his final deed
had been done:

> On Monday afternoon he was called to his surgery. On re-
> turning home he was taken ill, and passed away in a chair.

In Dolycwrt, Dr Penn assumed overall responsibility virtually overnight. Times were now both strenuous and arduous,
because Dr Gibbin's terrific experience and expertise, and his
knowledge and command, were sorely missed. There were
enormous gaps to fill besides Dr Gibbin's close companion-
ship and extraordinary presence, which Dr Penn could not
forget.

Now, just a close-knit two man team, Dr Merrell became
a partner in the practice. At times like this, locums such as
Dr Penn's college friend and second row rugby partner, Dr
David Boyns, were invited to lend their support. This helped
enormously, but, faced with a growing list of patients and
an expanding workforce at the milk factory next door, no
time was wasted in applying to the Health Authorities for

assistance. Filling the available vacancy was Dr Malcolm Holding, who has remained in Whitland as a well-known and respected figure ever since. In the height of the busy summer period, while local farmers were harvesting their crops, Dr Holding arrived, on August 1ˢᵗ 1962, having made the long journey from Gloucester Royal Hospital. As a schoolboy, Dr Holding had been brought up at Eltham, South East London. In the heavy onslaught of continued German air raids in the early 1940s, a bomb landed in the back garden of his family home. He was promptly evacuated to the delightful Gloucestershire setting of Newnham-on-Severn, aged just ten. After attending Lydney Grammar School, and later the National School of Medicine, Cardiff, he qualified in 1956. The following February, Dr Holding became a House Officer at Glangwili Hospital, Carmarthen, in the days of the Nissen Huts. He next moved to Bridgend Hospital, for 18 months of midwifery and paediatrics before returning to Carmarthen for two more years. He then transferred to Gloucester Royal Hospital before starting general practice at Whitland.

When Dr Holding was asked about the early days, he said that he had visited Whitland to make domiciliary calls whilst in Carmarthen. It was when working in Glangwili that he saw Dr Penn for the first time, and Dr Gibbin, too, because they were both regular visitors when their patients were admitted. During his first stay at Glangwili, he lived in the residential quarters of the old Priory Street Hospital, the scene of Dr Creswick Williams' great work in 1890. At the time, this hospital also handled the telephone switchboard for Glangwili.

One afternoon, Dr Holding stepped in to man the phones. The usual telephonist was away, and no one else was available. The Nissen Huts had been put in place by the American soldiers in the Second World War, before the site became a civilian hospital. When Dr Holding returned for his second term, he arrived at an entirely different Glangwili, new and thoroughly modern, with excellent facilities. Towy, Teifi and Cleddau Wards were open, while the Nissen Huts initially remained for X-Ray and other functions.

On his first day at Dolycwrt, Dr Holding remembers turning into the driveway of the surgery. Mr Jack Williams, a former signal man at Whitland's West Box, was helping with the filing, and in the waiting room was a chapel bench for patients to sit on. Calls were charted on a large black board provided by Dr Gibbin, and there were some old medical instruments in the small cellar, where medical samples were also kept. During the first few days, he was taken around the country surgeries at Tegryn, Crymych, Hermon, and Llanglydwen, and he remembers being held up at Penclipen railway crossing. It was all very different for Dr Holding coming from Gloucester, he was struck by the remoteness of the practice:

> I was driving a grey Morris Minor at the time, and I remember George had a sporty Triumph Herald. He was thoroughly modern in those days, being one of the first doctors to set up a radio-phone system, so that the surgery could reach him when on visits. The aerial was on the roof of Dolycwrt, but, being down in the valley, the reception was limited. We later moved all the equipment to a higher location and this worked well. When I arrived, Dr Merrell was in his last year. He was very popular and spent a lot of time with the patients, but he wanted a change and left to take up a Health Board appointment.
>
> I enjoyed being taken around the practice by George and I always felt that there was a real sense of occasion at the country surgeries. I remember the early years at

Clynderwen. It was like a scene from *Under Milk Wood*. There would be plenty of onlookers – pretending to brush the street, or to clean the windows – but they were really watching to see who was walking into the surgery. In the country we sometimes had to walk across fields to get to patients. Before I arrived in Whitland, I thought that St Clears was the end of the world, but the country scene soon grew on me.

Medicine had learnt a lot from the war experiences and things had progressed since the N.H.S. in 1948. The old Nissen Huts were surprisingly efficient, clinically clean and comfortable, usually with a fuel burner in the middle of the ward, with a long vertical escape flue straight through the ceiling. The new Glangwili was a highly modern hospital. We had a Royal Visit for the big day in 1959 and George was there taking photos. There is a picture of him in a souvenir booklet watching the opening ceremony. Tuberculosis was rampant in the 1940s and 1950s, but a lot of hard work was put into combating it. Various measures were introduced, one being streptomycin, which was very effective. We used to carry out all sorts of minor operations at Dolycwrt – sebaceous cysts, moles, sutures, lacerations, lipomas, foreign bodies. We would always be patching up the rugby boys with stitches, too.

Before I arrived in Whitland, I preferred football. As a child I had watched Charlton at the Valley, and in medical school I sometimes went along to see Cardiff City. But this all changed when the rugby players turned up at Dolycwrt on a Saturday night. I remember shortly after I arrived, we needed a new operating table. George found one at a private hospital in Bristol. A lorry from Mansel Davies and Son, the local haulage company, went to fetch it, and we had to find a few more strong men from the Dairies to bring it into Dolycwrt. It was very heavy and awkward to move.

Around that time, Mr Dormer held a dental surgery at Dolycwrt once a week. Dr Gibbin had extended the practice in his day, taking on patients around the Crymych area. So, we had a lot of travelling to do; they were busy times, but it was all very enjoyable at Dolycwrt.

It was only a month later, in the early Autumn of 1962, that one of the saddest events to take place in the Taf valley was also to impact upon Dolycwrt Surgery. This was the closure of the Cardi Bach railway. To this day, people say it should not have happened and, certainly, its execution should not have been so final. The tracks that had been laid after years of tireless work were ripped up at the first opportunity, and the land was sold. In one fell swoop, it committed to memory all that John Owen had heroically achieved, when pioneering its early beginning in 1873, before Dr Creswick Williams had even entered medical school.

Dr Holding told me that he remembered the day, it was Saturday September 8th 1962, when hundreds of people packed on to the train to Cardigan for the last time. Then, overnight, the passenger service ended, and a bus took over. Freight continued for a while longer but, this, too, ended in May 1963.[55] Soon the track lifting was in full swing – completed in July 1964 – and the land was sold in many parts. It was as clinical as that.

In the period leading up to closure, there was heightened interest, as can be expected, with public meetings. Speaking out in one of these events was Dr Penn. He introduced himself as a doctor and parish councillor from Whitland, whose practice was covered by the Cardi Bach. He mentioned

55 *The Whitland and Cardigan Railway*, M. R. C. Price, The Oakwood Press.

that this railway had always had a great bearing on medical practice in Whitland – a town born because of the railways, which had transported doctors, patients and medicines, as well as passengers and freight, for many years. It facilitated trading in the smaller villages along the line, and in Whitland itself.

He mentioned that the country surgeries, purposely located along the northern halts, testified to the great importance of the line but stressed that there was still the need to link patients to the main medical base, Dolycwrt, in Whitland. Acknowledging advancements in motoring, he explained why there was a place for road and rail transport. He considered the impact of closure on future trade, and he called for an official local committee – not in London – to review passenger activity.

This time, Dr Penn's words fell on deaf ears. In the circumstances of Dr Gibbin's passing, and now being senior partner, he had no time to mount one of his more serious railway campaigns, such as fighting to save the main line to Tenby and Pembroke Dock, which was a major victory. Losing the Cardi Bach, near to his small surgeries, was like having Dolycwrt's front consulting room bombed. It hurt him and the practice; no doubt, it would have hurt his forbearers, too. From that moment, Dr Penn would not let such a recurrence take place, at least, not without a fight. While he realised that a failing business could not forever be subsidised, he craved for the opportunity to do something about it. To him, the big 'carve-up' was unacceptable. As far as railway closures were concerned, he was prepared for battle.

In the aftermath of all of this, many people shared an unbelievable passion for the Cardi Bach. Now, almost fifty years later, it is still the same. People cannot let go of the special memories. One of Whitland's well-known railwaymen, who regularly worked on the line, is Les Rowlands. It is Les who fainted when Dr Owen was buried in 1937, and it is Les who saw Sir Winston Churchill at the Station Square in 1941. He was a fireman on the Cardi Bach, and his grandfather before him was a guard.

Les was aware that Dr Penn viewed the Cardi Bach's closure as a personal affront to the values he wanted to uphold at Dolycwrt: tradition, continuity, accessibility and convenience for patients. Les shares some of his memories about the old line, with a mention, also, about the doctors:

The small surgeries were located near many of the station stops. Glogue and Rhydowen stations were near to Hermon, Tegryn and Glandŵr surgeries, and Crymych surgery was just a short walk from the station. But the best known surgery of them all was the Bont, in Llanglydwen. This is where people walked out of the pub and jumped aboard the Cardi Bach only fifty yards away. We had a lot of fun with the passengers at Llanglydwen. It was their favourite railway stop.

The Bont surgery was important for years, and all the doctors enjoyed going there. Dr Evans even helped behind the bar in his spare time. I called there one summer's day after work with a colleague. Dai and Lizzie, the owners, were turning hay in the field. Dr Evans was in charge. 'And what can I get for you, gentlemen?' he smiled as we approached the bar. He enjoyed the country life, the Bont being a good place to experience it.

The Dolycwrt doctors worked well with the railwaymen from the early days. They treated the men and taught First Aid, and their medicines left Whitland in a little basket – all sealed, labelled and ready for collection – on the four o'clock train. As a boy, I remember Dr Rowley Thomas, and although he had his own surgery, he teamed up with the Dolycwrt doctors when there were problems.

One night, I was in the Yelverton Hotel, Whitland, when one of the locals was complaining bitterly of toothache.

'Rowley's in the next bar,' said one of them.

So, in he came, a lovely man, kind; he had a mischievous smile.

'Give him some whisky,' said Rowley in a loud voice, 'Send him into the back room, and fetch me some pincers.'

I remember there was a bit of shouting, but Rowley soon had the tooth out. Then he would make us laugh.

On another day, I cycled to see him at Parke. I went down the long lane to his house. Rowley was sitting in the chair; a shawl was wrapped around him. I think he had been sleeping.

'My father sent me up to see you,' I said.

'Who's your father?' he replied.

I told him. I needed a certificate that day. He reached over. His pad was near him on the stool.

'Half a crown,' he said. This was before the National Health Service. Doctors had to charge then.

Whitland inherits Parc Dr Owen

FOLLOWING 1963'S COLD winter of snow and ice, and the opening of Whitland Rugby Club at Caxton House in September, attention turned to a generous gift that had been given to the town. This refers to the vast acreage of the park, once known as the Recreation Field, then as the Town Field, before its name was changed yet again.

As earlier mentioned, Dr Owen, who lived and worked in Dolycwrt for twenty-four years, was known for his charitable nature and, following his early passing in 1937, his family added to his kindnesses by allowing the town to use the Recreation Field (as it was called in his day). Whilst it was years later that a Trust Deed committed everything to print, his sister Mrs Mildred Morris, as Grantor, conveyed the playing fields to the town people. This was given in ... 'The memory of her brother, Dr William David Owen, of Dolycwrt, Whitland' and, from this time onwards, the large playing-area was affectionately known as Parc Dr Owen.

In order to raise money for the park's upkeep, with grass to cut and hedges to trim – and to enhance the facilities, such as providing new swings and roundabouts for the children – a new Entertainment Committee for Parc Dr Owen was established. The first entry in the minute book explained the Committee's purpose: to make arrangements for a full week of money-making functions, which was to be called Parc Dr Owen Week:

At a meeting held on Wednesday 27th May 1964, it was decided to hold these functions from Sunday 30th August to Sunday 6th September. The members chosen to form this Sub Committee were: Dr G. K. Penn, Mr Harold Harries JP, Mr F. Merriman, Mr Eric Thomas, and Mr F. Jefferies.

From these early beginnings the concept of the (later named) 'Whitland Week' was born, something that has given immense pride, delight and entertainment to the locals ever since. Dr Owen's family were, no doubt, extremely proud to return to Whitland at the end of August to attend some of the events which made up the final programme. These included cricket and rugby matches; a Cheese and Wine social evening at Whitland Abbey; a Grand Celebrity Concert at the Grammar School, a Talent Competition in the Festival Hall, and a United Thanksgiving Service at Tabernacle. But the main attraction was the Carnival and Fete in the park, and it has remained the biggest event of the week ever since.

It was about a year later that Dr Penn took over as secretary – an office that he was to hold on to for sixteen years, until 1981 – with regular meetings now continuing at Dolycwrt Surgery. Besides being more convenient for Dr Penn, and other members, Dr Penn was by now very attached to the old building. He appreciated its special atmosphere, knowing that it was appropriate for Parc Dr Owen committee meetings to be held in Dr Owen's former surgery-home. He was proud to support the park, following the traditions already set by his predecessor, and he revelled in the creativity of organising events which brought happiness and togetherness to the people of Whitland.

There is no doubt that the Week's entertainment galvanised the small town that was still growing in many ways. This beautiful and prestigious park, situated near the milk factory, railway station, schools, surgery, pubs and shops, gave Whit-land a strong core. From the beginning, it had been intended that other organisations be fully involved, and, to everyone's credit, this is exactly what happened. Indeed, Dolycwrt's doctors, nurses and patients all played their parts in supporting Whitland Week over the years, while participating in the carefree occasions of free-flowing fun and entertainment, which visitors from far outside the town also came to enjoy.

Year after year, there were new attractions: mohicans, death riders, parachutists, rodeos, jalopy races, wrestling, and fashion shows, besides the more usual concerts, tug-of-wars, and traditional community events. Through the services of the Daubney Variety and Gala Agency, in Sheffield, huge celebrities came to the town. These included *Coronation Street*'s T.V. stars Julie Goodyear (Bet Lynch), Bernard Youens (Stan Ogden), Jean Alexander (Hilda Ogden), and Pat Phoenix (Elsie Tanner). All of this was serious entertainment, and behind it was some serious work. Like Dr Penn, who dedicated his summer fortnight to the 'Week,' Peter Wills, a schoolteacher, sacrificed his school holidays, having joined the committee in the early years.

Peter, whose late Aunty Vi (Violet Smith) used to remind him about the vicar's wife cycling to St Mary's Church on a penny-farthing bicycle, enjoyed the meetings at Dolycwrt, also remembering Dr Penn being called away occasionally to urgent visits. But, as part of the hard-working committee, he shared a passion for Whitland Week with his colleagues, and this was to last for many years.

When Peter spoke about the old days, he reeled off a number of stories. One of his favourites concerned the wrestling event. This was a huge attraction and, on the night, the marquee was packed with people who, having paid, were sat eagerly awaiting the action. In the middle was a big space for the ring, and this was to be erected by the wrestlers when they arrived. But, with the clock ticking away, it appeared as a gaping hole, and there was no sign of them. Outside, in Market Street, Peter remembers Dr Penn's words,

'Peter, if these wrestlers don't turn up soon, you and I had better head for the hills.'

To say that these were worrying moments is an understatement. Only minutes later, coming round the Fisher's Corner was a big removal van. As it approached, the driver wound his window down and called out,

'Hoi mate, is this Whitland?'

As Peter answered, his prayers were answered, too.

'Then where's the wrestling, mate?'

The entire team and back-up men were in the van. Soon everyone clambered out, and the ring was assembled, and the wrestlers were changed. But before the action began, they wanted to identify someone in the front row for some fun.

'And who are you looking at, you miserable . . .?' snarled the giant wrestler as he pointed towards a local character in the front row. That was all it needed: up he shot from his seat, arms waiving, fingers pointing and fists clenched, as he threatened the wrestler, twice his size, but from the spectator side of the ropes. The crowd went wild with excitement. It was a riot. And the wrestling had not even begun. Peter explained:

We used to have some terrific times during Whitland Week. That act at the beginning of the wrestling was the spark that ignited the entire evening. But before the wrestlers arrived, George and I were on tenterhooks. There was a huge crowd of people sitting in the marquee, having travelled miles that night. Like the rest of us they were beginning to get impatient. I can tell you George and I breathed a sigh of relief when the wrestlers poured out of that van. Things were getting tense.

I remember on another occasion, we held an 'It's a Knockout' competition in the Town Field. It took an enormous amount of preparation, and we advertised it well, with good prize money. That day we had nearly three thousand people in the park. This is the most that I can remember.

The Blue Stars Parachute team gave a spectacular display. Everyone remembered that day. Then we had the Mohicans going through fire, and the International Death Riders launching their motor bikes into the air – clearing a very long line of cars. It was all unforgettable entertainment. One year we invited the popular British group the Moody Blues; then we brought down a talented band of young ladies called the Dagenham Girl Pipers. They were given lodgings in the town, and then made a grand entrance into the packed marquee, taking everyone by surprise. They were magnificent.

We used to have some great personalities and celebrities in our carnivals, too. We invited Delme Thomas in the early 1970s, a British Lion. Of course, the *Coronation Street* stars were great fun. They travelled a long way and usually stayed overnight. Before the carnival, we treated them to a nice lunch in a local hotel. On the occasion of Jean Alexander's visit – her screen name being Hilda Ogden – she stayed with Willie Richards, at the Fishers Arms. On the Friday night, she was busy pulling pints behind the bar. The local people loved her. We had some wonderful fun in those days.

And every year we reminded everyone that our programme of events was for the purpose of maintaining and enhancing the park. It had been a wonderful gift from Dr

Owen's family. During many years at Dolycwrt, Dr Owen's countless good deeds had enriched the lives of people in the town and its surrounding areas. It is so important that memories of the great doctor live on.

Dolycwrt shares the Good Times of the 1960s

WHITLAND IN THE 1960s was a booming town full of enterprise with opportunities galore. Besides the railways, the milk factory stood tall and bright, a beacon of employment without equal for miles around offering a huge range of work from basic cleaning and clerical duties to the more specialised laboratory and food processing functions. The huge fleet of lorry drivers collecting milk across west Wales was just a small arm of its enormous operations, which saw traders of all description, including blacksmiths and tinsmiths, arriving daily at the site only a few doors away from Dolycwrt Surgery.

Mair Evans moved to Whitland from Clynderwen, where she used to visit Dr Gibbin in the small weekly surgery at Cambrian House. Mair remembers these busy times:

> We used to see crowds of people working in Whitland, bringing trade to the shops, cafes and pubs. Wilson and Merriman were selling tractors, Lionel James was selling new cars, and there were petrol pumps at every turn. The centre of Whitland was a hub of activity, and sitting in the middle of it all was our little surgery.
>
> I have wonderful memories of Dolycwrt, where I used to wait – sometimes for hours – for Dr Penn. He was often called out from surgery on emergency calls, so everyone would relax in the waiting room, happily watching television or reading magazines. No one seemed to mind; it was comfortable there. We all knew that we could have a

good talk to Dr Penn when he arrived.

In the early 1960s, when he had the help of Dr Merrell, we could hear the radio system making noises in the background. This was shortly before Dr Holding arrived. The country surgeries were well attended, including the one in Clynderwen. There were chairs in the passageway for us to wait, while the doctor used the front room.

There was a lot of pressure on Dr Penn following Dr Gibbin's sudden death. Dr Gibbin was well known in the area, and had been in Dolycwrt for approaching thirty years. At the time, Dr Roland Lewis was also practicing in Whitland, working from King Edward Street. I used to see him passing up North Road, and he had his own little surgeries in the district.

Nurse Hopkins had become well established in the area by now. She would often be seen going in and out of Dolycwrt. She was also in and out of the chemist shop, too. As a nurse and midwife, she often travelled into the countryside so she used to drop-off medicines and tablets on her rounds. This is how I remember the old days of Whitland, when people were helping each other all the time.

Dr Holding explained that his sister-in-law, Hazel Thomas – today Hazel Scrivener – was a welcome addition to the team. She was the first full time receptionist employed at Dolycwrt. Hazel set up new filing systems, answered the phones, and generally looked after patients when they called. Dr Holding explained:

Hazel also became efficient with the radio system. She used to page George and me as 'Dol-Doc-1' and 'Dol-Doc-2.' Hazel manned the phones and she used to bring the patients in to see us in the consulting rooms. Surgeries were busy then throughout the day. Of course, there were no appointments, and patients could choose when they wanted to call. Surgery hours were three times a day after meals, a little bit like the instructions on the medicine bottles. Surgeries began at 9.30, 1.30 and 5.30. But as a rule, people chose to come to the last surgery, which often ended late in the evening.

When Hazel left Dolycwrt in the late 1960s, Anne Griffiths – today Anne Bowen – replaced her. Anne was well known in Whitland as Mr Vivian Griffiths' daughter. He ran the chemist at Medical Hall with Eddie Evans, and Anne's family lived behind the dispensary for over fifteen years. Anne remembers the day, in 1969, she started work in Dolycwrt:

> I remember thinking . . . what have I let myself in for? It was so different from my previous work. There were so many things to remember, and I didn't know patients' names. They knew me as the chemist's daughter, and I had known them all my life, but how was I to ask them their names?
>
> But things improved, and I really enjoyed the variety: answering the phones, doing paperwork, filing documents into the cubby-hole system, writing repeat prescriptions for the doctors to sign, and welcoming the patients. There was always plenty to do.
>
> The surgery had its own special atmosphere: small rooms, narrow doorways, and a long passageway – and I remember we once took a look into the old loft. Amongst a supply of medicine bottles were some cricket pads and boots. I believe these may have belonged to Dr Gibbin.
>
> We enjoyed a happy atmosphere, and, just before my wedding, I booked two days holiday. I didn't mention that I was getting married, but one morning all three of the doctors were waiting for me, saying that they had changed

their minds; I couldn't have the time-off. They were smiling; someone had told them my news.

Down the road in Medical Hall, my father worked hard in the chemist shop. It was always busy, and we received deliveries in the big Winchester bottles. Occasionally, one would break, and there would be a big mess, and an even bigger smell. We often saw the doctors chatting at the dispensary, and people called with their prescriptions at all hours, sometimes late at night. But my father didn't seem to mind. Work was more informal in those days, and Dolycwrt was much the same.

Next door to the old chemist is today's longest-serving business in the town, M. L. Davies, the hardware and furniture store. Today it is run by Mary Pearce, whose parents took over the shop in 1950:

I can still see the antique cabinets, and beautiful old medicine bottles, most with colourful labels. It was a wonderful old-style chemist: small, compact. It had a wooden counter, and generous shelving, and it was always busy; Dr Penn and Dr Holding would come and go on their travels, as people arrived all day long.

Whitland was so lively in those days. Crowds flocked into town on mart days, side-stalls packed the streets on fair nights, and the pavements were full at Christmas time. I remember the men coming out of the pubs at half past four on Christmas Eve, suddenly remembering that they had to take a present home. They were merry, full of good cheer, and we often helped them choose a gift.

Next door would be no different as last-minute shoppers crowded inside. Then patients arrived from Dolycwrt, on their way home from surgery. The dispensary was just like Dolycwrt, it seemed to be open all the time.

Dr Allen arrives in Time for
the Investiture Celebrations

A T THIS SAME TIME, in the late 1960s, Dr Roland Lewis made his move to Narberth, having built up a successful practice at King Edward Street. He was missed in the community, having given years of service, and, at this juncture, many of his patients moved across to the Dolycwrt practice. Now a third partner was needed, at a time when medicine was advancing in leaps and bounds. More than 250 miles away, in the small town of Belper, near the Derbyshire coalfields, Dr Roy Allen was looking to move to west Wales. His father-in-law, Mr Leslie Busby, had built a bungalow in. Whitland and while visiting his family Dr Allen had got to know Dr Holding, next door. Following a very long journey from Derbyshire to Whitland for an interview, he later started at Dolycwrt on January 1st 1969.

Dr Allen was born in West Ham, London, but moved with his family to Barking, Essex, at four years of age. He attended Dagenham County High School, where he enjoyed sports, especially football. He was in good company: Sir Alf Ramsey and Terry Venables, two distinguished England managers, were both Dagenham boys. At the Royal Free Hospital, King's Cross, London, he qualified as a doctor in 1960. On route, he attended the Royal College of Surgeons where, in 1887, Dr Creswick Williams had also been examined. Dr Allen remembers a special ceremony. Upon hearing his name called out – meaning he had passed – he stepped aside to join other successful candidates, before being summoned to sign the register and to swear by the Hippocratic Oath.

Dr Allen undertook his first few hospital jobs in London, before moving to Derby City Hospital in 1962. He then entered a small partnership, where many of his patients worked in the nearby mines, whilst others shared with him a love of Derby County Football Club. In those days, Derby County played at the Baseball Ground, a compact old stadium that buzzed with atmosphere. They were a formidable team then, just before the truly great days of Brian Clough and Peter Taylor. Derbyshire was delightful. The industrial areas were surrounded by rich green countryside, and there were big cities all around. But a 'Whitland Welcome' was waiting in the hillsides, and Dolycwrt would be his next stop:

I remember my first two weeks. Dr Penn insisted on taking me round to meet everyone. It was very formal, but in Wales people appreciated this; it was the country way. The Branch Surgeries were all very interesting, each very different. The 'Bont' was lively. I remember being caught up there in the snow once, probably a few years after I arrived. One of the locals took me down a farm lane on a tractor, with the front-end-loader clearing the snow. It was the only way through. Afterwards, I was taken to the Bont surgery, freezing cold and soaking wet. The patients were waiting, but the landlord made a nice hot dinner and sat me in front of the glowing fire. Then he called the patients in. That's how it was; everyone was kind.

When I arrived in Whitland, the chemist was still at the old premises, Medical Hall. We were at the end of an interesting decade of medicine. We had seen some amazing breakthroughs. Both kidney and heart transplants had taken place, and test tube babies were being talked about. Steroids were playing a bigger part, and a far wider selection of drugs was available from the pharmaceutical companies. We had already entered into an era of more pronounced scientific medicine, involving detailed clinical checks, preventative measures, targets and incentives, too.

Everyone referred to the 'swinging sixties,' and this was true. Away from medicine, so much was happening. We had the Beatles, and the far greater T.V. coverage had changed people's lives. We saw better roads, improved cars, more modern aeroplanes; it was all taking off. I remember waiting up with my family one night when Neil Armstrong was landing on the moon. These were unbelievable days and in the middle of it all England won the World Cup. I happened to be in London that weekend. Although I didn't see the game, I could not miss the excitement. We were all thrilled.

Dr Allen remembers Whitland's Investiture celebrations in 1969, the year that he arrived in Dolycwrt. Considerable preparations had been made in the town to organise a varied programme of events, which culminated in the visit of Prince Charles as the Prince of Wales. Everybody enjoyed the celebrations, giving this important royal occasion the respect it deserved. As ever, the Memorial Hall Committee was well ahead of the game: preparing for Prince Charles' visit well in advance, as confirmed by the minutes of the annual meeting held on Friday June 13th:

> Members of the committee had been requested to attend a short meeting after the A.G.M. to discuss the renovations needed before Investiture Day, and also the visit of H.R.H. Prince Charles.

The celebrations began with a United Divine Service that was held at Tabernacle Chapel on Sunday June 29th 1969, presented by Danny Stephens. Following this was a dance on Tuesday July 1st for both children and adults. The next day, an afternoon of sports and tea was scheduled for Parc Dr Owen, while later in the evening a variety concert took place at the Grammar School. The popular local group Perlau Taf featured with supporting artists.

On the morning of Thursday July 3rd the Prince of Wales began his busy day with a Service of Dedication, held at St David's Cathedral, commemorated by a rather grand programme, with a detailed Order of Service. Enjoying the splendour of this packed royal occasion in the delightful little Pembrokeshire city, were Dr and Mrs Penn, courtesy of an invitation from Her Majesty's Lieutenant for the County of Pembroke, the Honourable Hanning Philipps, MBE, JP.

Later that same day, the Prince of Wales made his way across the county, through Haverfordwest and into Carmarthenshire. Awaiting his arrival in Whitland's Market Street, besides a blaze of colourful flags and bunting, were the excited people of the town. As he stopped outside the Memorial Hall, and left his car to meet local dignitaries, he was looking smart, young, happy and relaxed. He was waving and smiling, as everyone gave him a hearty cheer.

The streets were packed that hot summer day, and among the hundreds of school children lining the streets with small flags, were pupils of my class, too. We had a little song for our royal guest, which had been well-rehearsed and perfected. For this reason the tune is still familiar after all these years – although it is Eilir Blethyn, former caretaker at Dolycwrt Surgery, who remembers the words:

Among our ancient mountains,
And from our lovely vales,
Oh, let the prayer re-echo
God Bless the Prince of Wales.

People were seen balancing on boundary walls during this fleeting visit, while others looked down from upstairs windows. For those who even climbed onto nearby garage rooftops, they would have seen the Prince enter a different car at the Memorial Hall, before he continued his journey to Carmarthen. As he passed Dolycwrt, where the children's singing was clearly heard, the crowds reached out to catch an all-important last glimpse of the visitor, before he disappeared round the Fisher's (Arms) corner. Leon and Margaret Thomas, the surgery caretakers, always took pride in the premises. They would have given the doctors' plate an extra polish that day and, like everybody else, they would not forget the visit of the Prince of Wales to our town.

The Doctors share some
Glorious Rugby Memories in the 1970s

I F WHITLAND'S Dr Rowley Thomas had lived to see the
1970s, he would have been an even prouder man. The
British Lions, with almost half their touring party being
Welsh, did the unthinkable: travelling to New Zealand and
winning a Test Series. More importantly, no less than seven
of these star performers were from London Welsh, the club
Rowley helped to found way back in 1885.

This unforgettable feat was to be the start of many
glorious rugby moments of the 1970s, both on the local
stage in Whitland and nationally. As Christmas arrived
in 1971 Doctors Penn, Holding and Allen were feeling the
excitement of a major rugby clash to be staged at Parc Dr
Owen on Saturday December 27th. The local club was to host
the might of Pontypridd Rugby Club in the National Knock-
out Cup competition. The visitors, an established first class
team in the old Welsh Merit Table league, boasted seasoned
campaigners and well-known names, and were expected by
many to ease to victory. They were in for a shock.

Brian Harries, one of the club's stalwarts, was controlling
the game at outside-half. He told me that the team was ready
for Pontypridd. Some of the rules of the game had altered
earlier in the season, which made the game faster. Whitland
was full of good runners and, with the new laws suiting
Whitland's fast and open style of play, many teams were given
a surprise that year.

The build-up to this fixture was different. We did some extra training in the sand dunes at Pendine. The match was two days after Christmas, and we went training on Christmas day. Certainly there was no drinking, nothing at all. Our focus was on Pontypridd: a top side. But our coaches Peter Wills and Graham Thomas had done their homework. We met before-hand at the Yelverton Arms to discuss tactics. When the day arrived, we were prepared.

There was a big crowd at Parc Dr Owen that afternoon. Most people were in the middle of their Christmas break, and came down to watch. The television cameras were also there. I remember the excitement and noise. The atmosphere fired us on. We all played really well, but the match ended as a draw.

During those earlier years of the National Cup, we had to spin a coin for a winner. Dennis John, Pontypridd's captain – a fine scrum-half during the same era as the great Gareth Edwards – won the toss for Pontypridd. It was a cruel way to lose. In the dressing room afterwards, there was disappointment, but also immense pride, because we had deserved to win. It was a big day for the Club.

Dr Holding, who used to be club medical officer, would have seen the headline in Pembrokeshire's *Western Telegraph* the following week 'Toss of a Coin Robs Whitland.' He was also one of the crowds that day, experiencing the moment when the home team were so close, and yet so far, from winning. But, at least, all the players survived the rigours of the match, and Dolycwrt had a quiet Saturday evening, allowing everyone to enjoy the special atmosphere in the club house.

Gary Richards, who probably had the hardest task of all the Whitland players, having to mark Pontypridd's Tommy David – later a Welsh international, Barbarian and British

Lion – often had occasion to visit Dolycwrt during a long playing career, which brought his fair share of injuries:

> I can remember going to Dolycwrt after playing against one of the local teams. I had heard that Dr Penn didn't leave a mark with his stitching, and that day I had quite a deep cut on my chin. I remember Dr Penn chatting away and teasing me, and although he took his time, the job was soon finished, and I was back in the club. A few weeks later, there was no trace of the wound.
>
> I remember Dr Penn joining us for our end-of-season tour to Portsmouth in the early 1960s. We had a match or two to play, but the rest of the time we were enjoying ourselves. Dr Penn took his cine camera everywhere; he seemed to be taking pictures of most things, but when we went down to Portsmouth Harbour, to visit H.M.S. Victory, this worried the security guards who asked him to put his camera away.
>
> I was very grateful that Dr Allen was with us in a match at Milford Haven one day. I collided with an opponent, and broke my jaw. This was a serious injury, and Dr Allen took me all the way to hospital in Swansea. I was detained for more than a week.
>
> I had one more nasty injury when I broke my arm playing in a Whitland trial match. Dr Holding was on duty, and, after taking one look at my arm, he could see that it was broken. Again, I was soon heading for the local hospital.

It was during these years that Wales' glory team of the 1970s, was almost invincible. It was the era of regular Triple Crowns and Grand Slams, and most nations were in awe of the Welsh performances. There were great players, such as Gareth Edwards, filling every position in the team; and the coach of the side – the architect of this astonishing success

– was a gentleman who, in his working hours, visited doctors' surgeries. This is Clive Rowlands, who was often seen at Dolycwrt on official duty.

During Clive's era, players of this settled Welsh team turned out together, game after game. It is for this reason that the words of the late, but one-and-only, Bill McLaren CBE, can be recalled from memory – sometimes to be heard in Dolycwrt's waiting room during extended Saturday surgeries:

> And the ball is coming back on the Welsh side. It is Edwards to Barry John; John to centre Arthur Lewis; Lewis to Dawes – to J. P. R. Williams. My word, he's coming through like a train – out to Gerald Davies. Now he can motor … and … what a wonderful score for the Welsh!

Bill McClaren provided an injection of electricity to these matches. But, under the North Stand in the changing rooms, the sparks were flying with Clive Rowlands. He was the man who had our international rugby boys dancing on hot bricks. Whilst everyone savoured the powerful singing of *We'll keep a Welcome in the Hillsides,* just before kick-off, Clive was ensuring that the Welsh players felt ten feet tall. He was a man of focussed passion, sheer determination and patriotism, and all of these qualities were with him in Dolycwrt.

Roderick Richards was Secretary of Whitland Rugby Club for years before he became Chairman. During this time, he knew all three of the Dolycwrt doctors, appreciating their good work for the club. He explained:

> In Whitland we always tried to look after the players. We wanted them to enjoy their rugby, and having a good medical team behind us was important. This is where the doctors came in; they helped us in many ways.
>
> I remember Dr Penn being our president when we

bought Caxton House. Those were the days when we used to sit in the Captain's Cabin at the back of the club on a Saturday night drinking beer around a roaring log fire. Doc Penn, as I called him, used to watch many of our matches, standing near the half way line with his brown flat-cap. Then he'd cup his hands to his mouth and would shout-out loudly, 'Come on Whitland.' This would happen often. He was making his presence felt.

Dr Holding was our president in the later 1970s. By then his son, Michael, had developed into a fine wing three-quarter. He was a Schoolboys International, and Wales won the Triple Crown in his year, beating England, Scotland and Ireland. Dr Holding came along to our dinners in Werndale, Bancyfelin, and used to amuse us with his speeches. In fact he was very involved, travelling with us twice to Czechoslovakia. We had some tough matches to play on that tour, and he would be bandaging the boys when they came off the field.

Dr Allen followed him as medical officer. We appreciated all his services over a number of seasons. I remember him becoming a keen rugby man. He didn't miss many matches, and enjoyed travelling with the team.

And we were all fond of Dolycwrt. This is where I knew I could find the doctors when I had their international tickets. They all enjoyed the matches in Cardiff, when we used to meet up in the Model Inn. In the 1970s tickets were like gold; everybody wanted them. The doctors were no different, and they were always pleased to see me with tickets in my hands.

Patients jump aboard the Doctor's Train

BY THE 1970S, Dr Penn had become well known for his railway campaigns. Stung into action by the bitter loss of the Doctor's Train (the Cardi Bach) many years earlier, he had reacted to the massive railway cull of Great Britain by becoming Secretary of the West Wales Railway Action Committee. This was a determined group, who, in fighting rail closures, seriously locked horns with the railway authorities. They challenged the statements and statistics of the Railway Board and, in their heroic efforts to keep the lines open, turned their attention to promoting the railways in every way possible.

During a committed twenty year period, it is true that Dr Penn played a big part in saving many lines across Wales. He travelled extensively and fuelled a huge uprising amongst leading politicians and public authorities. Indeed, his name was well known far away in Westminster, where many Members of Parliament got used to receiving letters from Dr Penn, of Dolycwrt Surgery. Indeed Dolycwrt featured in some of his railway activities, one of which was a steam venture which today runs at Henllan, known as the Teifi Valley Railway. It was in the small waiting room, shortly after the patients had gone home, that the great minds came together at the beginning of this exciting new venture in 1974.

Dr Holding – who sometimes put patients at ease when giving injections, by saying, 'Don't worry, this won't hurt me' – used to regularly tease Dr Penn during these hectic days of railway activity. Raising his partner's spirits one day, he told Dr Penn that his efforts were paying-off:

'Yes, George, I was fishing on the River Taf last night – and the Tenby train came along. The passenger count had greatly improved.'

'Really, Malcolm?'

'Yes, there was a one hundred per cent improvement. There were two passengers on board.'

Of course, in truth, Dr Penn was making an enormous difference. Today's trains to Tenby are often crowded and, as roads everywhere become more congested, the dawn of an new transport era may soon be upon us, in line with Dr Penn's thinking. Certainly, he challenged Dr Beeching's activities, as Richard Parker quite rightly mentions in his recent book *The Railways of Pembrokeshire*:

> Credit must go to the West Wales Railway Action Committee, a group determined to keep the railways open. Led by the redoubtable Dr Penn of Whitland, whose remedies were far removed from those of Dr Beeching, but more beneficial to the patient.

Many of the Dolycwrt patients remember the excursion trips that Dr Penn personally – and his committee, collectively – arranged over the years on the scenic Heart of Wales Railway. This beautiful line which cuts through the middle of rural Wales was not itself free of closure threats. Dr Penn was anxious to demonstrate that it was well used, chartering special trains to take people to the Royal Welsh Show and the Shrewsbury Flower Show each year. Dr Penn would spread the word around in his practice area and many patients were quick to respond. Mair Evans remembers her mother, Sarah Ann Evans, being excited about her trip to Shrewsbury:

My mother was very happy to be going all the way to Shrewsbury by train. She travelled with three of her friends from Llandissilio, starting out from Whitland before seven o'clock. My mother had been to London and Scotland before, but she preferred to stay local. This was a long journey for her.

My mother often talked about the special atmosphere. Tea and coffee was available to everyone from the great big urns they kept in the guard's van, and drinks were taken to people's seats. Dr Penn walked the train back and fore, seeing that everybody was happy and Mrs Penn was also very sociable to everyone.

Mother enjoyed the scenery through Mid Wales, especially the Sugar Loaf Mountain region, and she liked to see the sheep and cattle in the fields. At Shrewsbury, she and her friends had a good look around the town. It struck her as being a beautiful place, with narrow alleyways and famous buildings like the Old Market Hall. She enjoyed the Shrewsbury Flower Show, too.

Before they came back, they had a meal somewhere near the station. By this time, Dr Penn had refilled the tea urns, so there were more drinks for everyone on the way home. Then they pulled into Whitland at about eleven o'clock. It was a thoroughly enjoyable day – and mother never forgot her ride on Dr Penn's train.

A Doctor's Secret –
and the Milk Factory Next Door

THE DOLYCWRT DOCTORS could, justifiably, be proud of their close neighbours, the milk factory. From its early beginnings as Merlin's Dairies, through and beyond the advancing years of Somerset and South Wales Dairy Company, then as the Wiltshire United Dairies, before becoming a pillar of the Unigate Dairies Group in the 1970s – it had been a major success story.

Dolycwrt, only a few doors away, witnessed its growth, seeing it slowly expand up the street and into the town becoming the employment oasis of an extended dairy community. In their time, each of the doctors saw at first hand its great advancements, starting with Dr Creswick Williams, at the beginning of its operations, when it was a galvanised shed at the old mart ground.

In Dr Owen's days, the solid tractor-like lorries were venturing into the country lanes to make early milk collections. In Dr Gibbin's time the factory had its own private railway siding to take the milk away. And when Dr Penn made his entry, automation had well and truly entered inside the factory gates.

As Dr Holding made his way to Dolycwrt in 1962, Whitland Creamery,[56] as it was often called, had become a huge concern with milk being collected from farms all over west

---

56 Conversation with Keith Thomas, former Manager of Whitland Creamery.

Wales. By now eggs, cheese, butter, dairy drinks, evaporated milk, powdered products and other food had also left the premises for more urban areas.

By the time Dr Allen arrived, the Old Rectory was a picture of prosperity, offering spacious and prestigious factory offices, set in beautiful award-winning landscaped gardens. The factory attracted a workforce from miles around, facilitating well over three hundred jobs. In these circumstances, commercial viability provided the green light of expansion as the perimeter of the factory site extended into the town.

This was to change the complexion of Whitland and it was to displease Dr Penn, too, despite him understanding that this was done in the name of prosperity and with every best intention. In truth, the factory premises had almost entered Dolycwrt's front door by now having replaced the demolished row of terraced houses adjoining the building. The serious expansion programme saw large towers and stacks standing beside the old surgery only yards away, peering down from a great height.

Although medicine continued to be practised undeterred, it did so in the shadow of a now colossal enterprise, which still continued to grow. Indeed, Dolycwrt was wanted next, but Dr Penn insisted his surgery was not for sale, and would not waver from this.

These were now very different days, as life raced away into a somewhat uncertain future. The old times of Dr Creswick Williams' horse and cart had long gone, and Dr Owen's vintage cars, too. There were no more milk churns, either, replaced by bulk tankers in this great new era. It is interesting to wonder what the old doctors might have thought about this progress. Dr Creswick Williams and Dr Owen had both known something interesting from their time, since buried under the past century of years. It concerns Whitland's Old

Rectory, and lays open the undeniable common ground shared by the doctors and dairymen over the years. When, in December 1891, the sad news of Dr John Phillips' death became known in the locality, people mourned his passing from far and wide. It was he who brought Dr Creswick Williams to Whitland as an assistant, but a short while earlier, while still serving the Narberth Union, Dr Phillips lived in its vicinity. In *The Welshman* of December 26th 1891, it is mentioned that, having obtained permission from the Local Government Board to move, 'He remained in Narberth until he had completed the building of his picturesque residence on his estate in Whitland.' Dr Phillips' residence was known as Tŷ Gwyn ar Daf.

Tŷ Gwyn ar Daf was also Dr Creswick Williams' address when he bought Dolycwrt in 1898. It was usual for assistants to lodge at the senior doctor's residence at that time but where exactly was it? Well, referring to an earlier plan of Whitland – when there were less houses, and the streets were noticeably narrower – situated across the road from the Fishers public house was a very special residence with a coach house nearby. Alongside it were the four bold words 'Tŷ Gwyn ar Daf'.

This was indeed the house built by the late Dr Phillips; it is where Dr Creswick Williams later lodged and it is where patients called to see the doctor in the 1890s. And, by a huge coincidence, it was later to become the administrative centre for the Whitland Creamery enterprise – still known as the Old Rectory, relating to yet another of its former functions in the past. This is also where Martha Jane Owen – grandmother of Yvonne Evans, mentioned earlier – remembers working with Dr Creswick Williams for the first time. Its delightful gardens, lawns, bushes, and pine trees, extend all the way down to the river where, until the late 1970s, just a mere stretch of the Gronw waterway separated it from Dolycwrt.

When I mentioned this to Lawrie Bowen, former personnel manager, and long term factory employee, he was amused. He knew that these two big players, having performed on Whitland's main stage over the years, had shared a close bond. Indeed, they have shared some of the territory as well. As Lawrie said:

> We were well looked after at Dolycwrt Surgery. Dolycwrt provided our factory doctors from the early years. But it was more than a doctor-patient arrangement: it was a close friendship, too.
>
> In the later years, Keith (Keith Thomas, manager of the enterprise) asked me to invite Dr Penn to hold a regular surgery on our site. This was held in our first-aid room, and it was very successful – because I was able to coordinate the 'surgery', so that everyone could get back to their work. This was also a good service for our staff. Sometimes people came in specially – even on their days-off – just to see the doctor.
>
> Over the years a first-aid expert trained our team to the standards of St John's Ambulance. This well-respected gentleman, was affectionately referred to as 'Bill Bandage'. He prepared everybody really well. Then the doctors came in to do the examinations.
>
> In the days of our factory surgery, Dr Penn and his colleagues couldn't do enough for people and we looked forward to seeing them at our social events. Dr Penn was also a regular visitor to the Dairy Social Club, where everybody wanted to speak to him. Sometimes people wanted a prescription too – and this was all in a day's work for Dr Penn.

Dr Hugh Lewis-Philipps
and the Changing Face of Whitland

I N 1976 a well known local doctor, who had done countless good deeds at Dolycwrt, died. Dr Hugh William Lewis-Philipps, JP (usually referred to as Dr Hugh Philipps), had often come to Dr Penn's rescue when work and outside commitments became pressing. On occasions when Dr Holding and Dr Allen were off duty, or away on holidays, Dr Penn, at his home in Whitland, would be heard saying to his wife,

'Now, how am I going to manage evening surgery and my follow-up calls, as well as getting to the railway meeting – and, of course, I am meeting Mr Thomas, the specialist, in the morning?'

Then, in his next breath, he had the answer,

'I know what I'll do Peggy, I'll ask Dr Hugh Philipps to stand-in for me for a few hours.'

When Dr Penn telephoned, the senior doctor needed no persuasion. He remained keen and active in medicine until the end. It was the perfect situation, and this happened often. In one of Dr Penn's diary entries, he described the time he was with Dr Hugh Philipps at a British Legion function in Cardiff, probably one of the few occasions when he was unable to help Dr Penn:

I had arranged to go to Llandaff Cathedral (and meet others from Whitland on a bus) for the fifty-year service of thanksgiving for the British Legion but I needed Dr Hugh

Philipps to stand-in for me. Unfortunately, he decided that he would like to go to the function himself. Therefore I could only go if I finished the morning surgery – if I was lucky … After the service there was a fall-in, which I joined, and we marched from Llandaff Cathedral to Llandaff Fields. Dr Hugh Philipps asked me to give him a lift to town so that he could meet his wife. Then, after collecting Peggy, we met Dr and Mrs Hugh Philipps at the Model Inn.

Dr Hugh Philipps served in the Royal Army Medical Corps and experienced active wartime duties. He became President of the Whitland and Llanboidy Branch of the, now, Royal British Legion and, according to the glorious tributes in his obituary, he was awarded the prestigious Gold Badge[57] for long service, as well as being a Justice of the Peace and High Sheriff of Carmarthen. Living in the delightful residence of Clyngwynne, Llanboidy, set on a bank among big mature trees, he could look out from his front bay-windows across the gentle lowlands to Llanboidy about a mile away.

At a family visit to Clyngwynne, Dr Penn was once shown a large silver cup that his senior colleague had won playing tennis. Clearly, he played to a high standard: even entering the Men's Singles tournament in Wimbledon in 1926.[58] Today, his name is recorded alongside the great players of Wimbledon's magnificent history. But, as for medicine, this gentleman was cast in the mould of the traditional old doctors, who, having emerged from Queen Victoria's reign, had seen the changing face of Whitland and of modern life.

In the later 1970s, Whitland was also saying goodbye to its Magistrates Court. Sister Eunice Hopkins JP, well known at Dolycwrt and in the practice area – was to notice a change.

---

57 The *Carmarthen Journal*, 24 December, 1976, Carmarthen Library Services.
58 The All England Lawn Tennis Club, Wimbledon.

This Court of Petty Sessions – formerly known as a Police Court – had taken place at the Memorial Hall since around 1928, although, in earlier times, these events were staged at Whitland Town Hall. In these two proud buildings, minor indiscretions – and not so minor ones, too – were given a full and proper hearing.

Sister Hopkins, one of five local magistrates sitting on a panel representing Carmarthen South, chaired by Con Harries JP, who runs a food store and catering firm in the town, explained that the team missed the greater informality of the local setting in Whitland, which everyone had grown to enjoy and respect. Again, time had moved on but, for Whitland, this was a sad loss. It was a case of another piece of treasured stone having been removed from its once impregnable 'town wall.'

There was no forgetting the disappearance of Black Bridge, either. Black Bridge was Whitland's gateway from the west – well remembered by many doctors over the years as being a nasty accident black-spot. It was replaced around the late 1970s by a more modern road structure.

Situated nearby, at that time, in the Westgate Transport Garage and Café was Whitland's Anne Jones. Anne told me that she remembers Black Bridge flooded so heavily that cars and lorries dropped down the other side into a lake of water. Anne explained:

> I can remember a number of accidents occurring at Black Bridge and, before the paramedics arrived, the local doctors were called to the scene. Black Bridge was positioned high on a bend. It was narrow, and had clearly been made for early-day traffic. Cars were steadily getting bigger, and I can remember both Dr Gibbin and Dr Evans having newer models, which were large vehicles, too.

Pengawse Hill, a little further west of Black Bridge, was also dangerous. When the hill was by-passed, everybody breathed a sigh of relief. Its long gentle bend made it impossible to overtake. I remember Dr Penn – who once had a bump at Pengawse Hill – talking about someone who had returned home from Australia. They had a wonderful journey, but the worst part was climbing Pengawse Hill, on their way back to Narberth!

In the days of my great aunt, who cycled daily to Clyngwynne mansion to work as a parlour maid, both Black Bridge and Pengawse Hill served the traffic well. But, in more modern times, new road structures were needed.

An Epic Journey in the Snow –
and a Patient's Call to Duty

THE WIND AND SNOW of January 1982 saw people freezing cold in Whitland's latest spell of severe weather. A thick white blanket covered the town and surrounding countryside, while further north on the higher ground nearer the Preseli Mountains the snow was deeper still. Strong blustery winds caused drifting, and roads became impassable. Often during conditions like this, Dolycwrt would be quiet, simply because it was not possible for doctors to travel far. However on this occasion, there was an urgent call to Efailwen.

Working alongside the surgery at Whitland Creamery that day was John Coaker, the factory transport manager. Understandably, John and his colleagues were experiencing major difficulties themselves, because the milk lorries simply could not get to the farms. John remembers Dr Penn arriving at the yard in the early afternoon looking for help. He had a serious journey to make. He needed a Landrover:

> 'There is no way that I can make it, John – but do you think we can get there in your Landrover?'
>
> 'Well, Dr Penn, the only way for us to know is to have a go,' was my reply. Eventually, we got as far as Llandissilio, but the snow covered the road up to the level of the hedges. It was impossible to continue, so we turned back: we had done our best.

Shortly afterwards in Whitland, Dr Penn spoke to the patient's family by telephone. Someone in Efailwen with a JCB was happy to clear a pathway through the snow if Dr Penn was prepared to follow behind in the Landrover.

Indeed, Dr Penn was determined not to waste a moment, setting-off, without delay, for a second time. On this occasion, he and his driver were accompanied by Dr Alun Hughes of Pontypool, a young man who was well known in Dolycwrt for doing locum work. After braving the elements for a few hours, they reached the Nant-y-Ffin Motel, Llandissilio, where they met Roy Thomas in his JCB:

> By the time we approached the Bush Inn, I turned to Dr Penn. 'Do you think it would be a good idea if we were to go inside to have something small to warm us up, doctor?' … 'John, I thought you were never going to ask.' Dr Hughes in the back seat was laughing. He was also giving his full approval; we were all so cold.
>
> We climbed back into the Landrover and continued for, what seemed like hours before calling on another of Dr Penn's patients for some hot tea. Then we progressed as far as Efailwen, until we simply could go no further. For about half a mile we walked along the hedgerows – it was never-ending – then we eventually arrived at the farm.
>
> Dr Penn's assessment of the situation was that the patient urgently needed to go to hospital. Phoning the medical emergency services, he was told that a Sea King helicopter was on its way from R.A.F. Brawdy. They had a map reference, and asked us to light a fire in the field because everywhere was white, with snow still falling. We gathered bales of straw in readiness – and waited.
>
> I remember hearing the helicopter, and seeing a powerful bright light shining out of the sky. It was so strange. In fact

it was eerie, like a scene out of *Star Wars*. Our fire was blazing by now, and the helicopter came down to land.

It was around daybreak the next morning when we appeared at Nant-y-Ffin Motel, still on the way back. We were tired, and frozen cold, and almost a beaten force. But Henry Thomas, the proprietor, came to our rescue by providing a full breakfast, everything that we could eat. And Henry refused to accept payment; this was his contribution to the operation.

When we eventually got back to Whitland, Dr Penn heard that the patient had been rushed to theatre, and was making progress. The helicopter mission had been vital: our journey through the snow most essential.

Today, Dr Alun Hughes is back in his homeland, where he is in medical partnership at Cwmbran. Now years later, the details of those biting-cold conditions have not escaped his memory. Summing-up this epic journey in the snow, he said:

The marvellous thing about it all was that Dr Penn knew someone who had a JCB. Dolycwrt was quiet that afternoon. There were few calls, and I went along for the ride.

I remember wanting to go back in the helicopter to the hospital but Dr Penn wasn't terribly willing. He was concerned about everybody's safety that night, including the helicopter pilots. Conditions were so bad.

We had an awful return journey. It was one thing getting there – when the adrenalin flowed – but quite another going back. When we arrived in Whitland, we went straight to the surgery to check our messages. Dr Penn and I were thrilled to see Dolycwrt again. Then we went home.

In the *Narberth & Whitland Observer* on January 22nd 1982 – where a photograph of icicles appeared on the front page, and the weather had a big bearing on the week's stories – a small headline read, 'Airlifted to Hospital.' In just a few brief sentences, it confirmed the good news that Dr Penn's patient was 'doing fine.'

It was all so different in the much warmer temperatures of the following summer of 1982. This was when Argentina's invasion of the Falkland Islands shocked the nation and dominated the news. As Britain responded with a Task Force expedition, Jonathan Dunford, a young patient of the Dolycwrt practice, was soon to be involved in the fierce heat of these battles.

He had followed his father, John Dunford, into the Armed Forces. It is John who earlier described Whitland during World War II, and it is John who later chauffeured Dr Penn for many years, allowing him to cat-nap during his all-action days. However, it was Jonathan, serving in the 1st Battalion of The Welsh Guards, who helped to recapture Port Stanley and the Falkland Islands. Having sailed out aboard the *Q.E.2* ocean liner, he was soon in the middle of serious combat. When he returned, Jonathan became Whitland's latest war hero to be welcomed home, and was presented with a commemorative watch from the local people in Whitland Town Hall.

A Look back in Time
as a Memorable Partnership Ends

W E WERE NOW experiencing the beginning of what was to be the end of a memorable partnership between Whitland's three doctors, Doctors Penn, Holding and Allen. As deadline-day drew nearer, no doubt thoughts of earlier days together may have sprung to mind. However, turning the clock back one hundred years – all the way to 1882 – a road surveyor by the name of Rees Davies was excited to see the completion of a fine piece of work. This was Prospect House, an important building, which was later to become a proud surgery, renamed Dolycwrt. But, at this time, it was a handsome residence, brand new, set in deep foundations, and ready to face all weathers and challenges that were to come.

It is again in *The Welshman*, that a wealth of information about Rees Davies, the Whitland road surveyor, has been found. He was a well-respected man, who served the local council for many years. He was possessed of great humour, and limitless energy, and he knew the composition of every piece of stone from all the little quarries and sites around Whitland, including those at Whitland Abbey, Cwmfelin, Egremont and Fforest. Indeed, to build Dolycwrt, this was essential. Only someone such as he could also bridge the gap separating the front dwelling of Dolycwrt from the entirely separate coach house at the rear. This happened some ten years after its construction, making Dolycwrt one big building, as proved by two official plans of the day.

Rees Davies was also the architect of at least two of the beautiful stone-built bridges which cross the river Taf and still charm our countryside today. At Login, he was the contractor. At Cwm Miles just down the road, he presided over the building of this other much-admired land mark. During the early years of the last century, he worked with Dr Rowley Thomas and the Whitland Rural District Council to see this bridge finalised and fully financed. But before it was certified, a load-bearing traction engine had to travel across this new structure. Whilst others checked their personal insurances, Rees Davies, as brazen as brass, and clearly confident about his work, offered to jump on board for the ride!

During this same era, he teamed up with Dr Creswick Williams on all manner of drainage, sanitary and flooding issues prevalent in the town and parish, with the sea wall at Pendine being another matter demanding his attention.

Buried near the entrance of Soar Cemetery, Rees Davies, a pastor's son, was given both a memorable funeral and an outstanding obituary in *The Welshman* of July 21st 1922. It described a large funeral, where roadmen of the Whitland Rural District Council were bearers, and condolences were publicly recorded from Dr Hugh Philipps, Dr Rowley Thomas, and Dr Owen.

Returning to the modern day, and nearing the end of 1982, the final touches were being applied to another prestigious building. It was very different to Rees Davies' work, but was one of a number of health centres now emerging all over the country, replacing the old-style doctors' surgeries. It was complete with spacious consulting rooms, reception and waiting areas, car parking facilities, modern equipment and facilities for meetings and clinics. These buildings represented the way forward in the modern era of medicine, and while smaller surgeries like Dolycwrt were still continuing, they were getting less in number and disappearing fast. For patients of the Whitland practice, changes were now afoot. Clarifying the situation at length was Dr Penn's intent in a letter dated December 1982: 'To Patients and Friends of the Whitland Practice.'

The letter explained that the new surgery conformed to a national trend for doctors to work from modern purpose-built accomodation, a trend that the Government supported. He mentioned, however, that Dolycwrt still appealed to him and that he would be staying there. When considering the size of the practice, extensive alterations were needed at Dolycwrt, or else new premises had to be found:

The main headquarters will be transferred from Dolycwrt in St Mary's Street to the new premises in North Road; and, in my opinion, the new building will prove to be really excellent for its purpose. Dr Holding and Dr Allen will be practising from the new premises and they may be having the help of another partner as well as junior doctors in rotation. For my part, I am grateful for the friendly agreement that I may be permitted to continue with a smaller practice in Dolycwrt.

In order that the arrangements are satisfactory and successful, the majority of patients should be registered with Dr Holding and Dr Allen in North Road. I therefore suggest that unless patients make special arrangements with me, they could accept the idea of being attached to the new surgery.

I am naturally very sorry that the partnership is splitting up but I hasten to point out that we are splitting up in an atmosphere of friendliness and cooperation which I trust will continue.

Also, I trust that the two practices will be helpful, one

to the other, in the future and that no resentment will be held towards anybody at any time regarding the decision made. In short, I hope we'll be as happy in the future as in the past.

With good wishes,

George K. Penn

Dr Holding remembers
a Special Rugby Triumph

A S CHRISTMAS came and went, the new year brought a very memorable event in the history of Whitland Rugby Club; Whitland Youth won the Welsh Youth Cup. This was something special to savour in the town, and a triumph to celebrate for years. In the final the local boys beat highly rated Cardiff in a match that was billed as a *David versus Goliath* contest. Dr Holding, whose son Michael would have played if he had not still been in school at the time (school boys not being allowed), explained:

> I remember I was working that weekend, but I was looking out for the result. It was a fantastic achievement for everyone connected with the team, and the club. I knew that the players had been together as a group for a number of seasons. In fact, they had performed successfully all along at different age levels.
>
> There were some genuinely talented players in the team, too, who I felt would progress far in senior rugby. It was not surprising that they did well in the competition. But beating Cardiff in the final was an outstanding achievement for Whitland.

When I spoke to team captain Chris Smith, some 27 years later, none of his immense pride regarding this terrific achievement had diminished. He remembers a closely fought game against very determined opponents. Every one of the players were heroes. Chris, a sharp scrum half, who was one of the quickest off the mark, went on to play for Whitland first team, with distinction. He told me that Whitland beat some tough opponents on the way, including Carmarthen Harlequins and a very motivated Treorchy team, on their home ground, in front of a big crowd of local supporters.

On the day of the final, three buses left the rugby club, one with the team and officials on board, and two carrying the home supporters. Many others travelled by car. The match took place at Ammanford, and Whitland's victory was masterminded by two of the club's all-time greats, Tony Bowen and Gary Richards, with Myrddin Evans – but known as Mervyn – being the Team Manager. Neil Jenkins was the open-side flanker, and remembers doing some serious running and tackling that afternoon:

> In the changing room underneath the old grandstand before kick off, we could hear a lot of movement above. We knew there would be good support, but when we ran out onto the field, we were overwhelmed by the large crowd. I think the whole of Whitland was there. Cardiff brought a big following, too, and I think they expected to win as a formality. But that day every one of our team played heroically until the final whistle.
>
> With only minutes to go, Cardiff were awarded a penalty. We were just a point ahead then, and the kick would have given Cardiff the lead. We held our breath. In the crowd was Reverend Nigel Griffin, vicar of St Mary's Church. I am told that he said a quick prayer at that point. We were very grateful he did. We needed that little bit of luck. The ball hit the post, bounced away and we cleared it to safety. Soon the match was over. Crowds ran onto the field. It was a wonderful feeling that none of us will forget.

When we arrived back in Whitland, we were treated as heroes. The Mayor of Whitland met us from the bus. It was Gerwyn Williams, another fine Whitland player in his day. We were given a barrel of beer, and later we were honoured with a smart blazer. In the Club Dinner that season, at Werndale in Bancyfelin, we had a team photograph in our blazers. It was a proud rugby moment for us all.

A Return to the Days of a Sole Practitioner

AS IT HAPPENED, the division of patients between Dol-ycwrt and the new medical centre, named Meddygfa Taf, suited everyone concerned, and this served to enhance the good spirit and cheer that prevailed as partnership days had drawn to a close. For Dr Penn, stepping back onto the lonesome trail, he would clearly miss both Dr Holding and Dr Allen. While patient care and surgery had always been his love – allowing him to spend as much time as possible with patients – he was the first to admit that neither administration nor organisation were his strongest points.

Both his colleagues were disciplined and highly modern doctors. Work rotas, accountancy issues, claim forms, and general practice management were comfortably absorbed into their working routines. They granted flexibility too, enabling Dr Penn to disappear to events, or meetings, in the middle of the week, or whenever. Of course, Dr Holding and Dr Allen were themselves busy in the community, both very popular and in demand. They had their own meetings, engagements, and presidencies, but they found that little bit of extra leeway, which Dr Penn appreciated so much.

Like all good partnerships, they each brought different values and strengths into the mix. They worked for each other, and the result had been an overwhelming success. When Dr Holding spoke about the time of the changeover, he admitted that he missed the old days and the old ways of Dolycwrt after twenty-one years, but likewise time had marched on:

At Dolycwrt, we had simply outgrown the premises. With more than six thousand patients, and limited facilities, we were facing difficulties. The waiting room could accommodate, perhaps, twelve at any one time; there were just two consulting rooms; there was no official reception area, and there was no space for private clinics. I know George was very disappointed, but he was realistic, too. He got involved in the early stages of the new building, and Roy and I hoped he would join us. We had the opportunity of acquiring a suitable piece of land in Whitland, with improved parking, but then one day, before we met the architect, George told us that he was going on his own. We must not forget that George had already been at Dolycwrt for nearly thirty years. He felt it was right to stay. He owned the premises, too.

In fact, I can remember the time – it was in 1967 – when he bought Dolycwrt. He came into work one morning and had heard that Mrs Mamie Gibbin, Dr Gibbin's widow, was about to sign over the deeds to the Dairies. Like a shot, George was on his way to see her in Saundersfoot; then to the estate agents; and then the solicitors. He was running around everywhere; he didn't do much work that day. The Dairies clearly saw Dolycwrt as part of their expansion programme; George had other ideas. It was a battle of minds. He was immensely proud of Dolycwrt. That day he was securing it as a surgery. Of course, when the new premises were being built, there were still single-handed practices around the country, but the more modern approach was clearly directing doctors and patients to the group practices – or health centres, as they were called.

I must admit, I missed George. He was a wonderful, caring doctor and he was an immensely loved character. I missed all his campaigns. I remember teasing him about his railway efforts; but, when we look back, he achieved a great deal, and I am proud of this. He fought to save many lines, and he was also the driving force behind the Teifi Valley Railway, a steam venture. The early meetings of this enterprise were held at Dolycwrt – in the mid-1970s – after surgery. I remember this well. As regards Whitland Week, George ran this in most respects. Every year, he reserved his fortnight's holiday for the activities, and he brought some very memorable and happy occasions to Parc Dr Owen. I was involved with the trustees for twenty years, so our paths often overlapped concerning the park. George threw himself into everything. He always had time for people; he would never let anyone down.

I remember the occasion of my mother's funeral at Newnham. Roy wanted to attend, so George was left to man the fort. We were at St Peter's Church, overlooking the River Severn, 120 miles from Whitland. Suddenly George and Peggy appeared. They did not stay long, because George had arranged a temporary locum, but they were there for us. Little stories like this sum-up George – and this was a long drive in those days, through the villages and towns – but he was doing this sort of thing for everybody. Clearly we kept in touch. We offered to include him in our night rota system, but he preferred to be independent. George was very close to his patients; for his sake, I believe they tried their hardest not to be ill at night.

Dr Allen was now living in the Old Vicarage in Llanboidy. He and his family had settled well in the community and enjoyed opening their garden for village fetes and occasionally firework displays. Like Dr Holding before him, having got to know the rugby boys and, having attended to their injuries, Dr Allen had been converted from football to rugby. He remembers Dolycwrt for its friendly atmosphere, and for being one of the few surgeries across the entire country with full-time residential caretakers. Looking back, he would miss it, but looking forward, he was excited about the new medical centre:

Having a modern, spacious establishment would make it easier for us to deliver all that was expected in those more modern times. I know that some traditional single-handed practitioners, like George, were really not prepared to move from their delightful old premises. George was not alone. But the new school of thought was gathering pace. At the time of the changeover, we used to have primary health care meetings at Dolycwrt. Everybody was welcome to attend – nurses, midwives, drug representatives. When we moved across to Meddygfa Taf, we continued them from there. George came along to these, at least to begin with. We would also see George, occasionally, at medical meetings. The Carmarthen Medical Society was strong and we had good talks. George liked to attend these.

We were all caught by the rugby 'bug', George, Malcolm and I. I had four committed years as medical officer. I thoroughly enjoyed travelling around with the team. One special match that stood out in my memory was against Pontypool. We played them in the Welsh Cup. In those days, the Pontypool front row was feared not only in Wales, but all over the world. They were all British Lions, and there were many other great players in their pack, and throughout the team. That day Whitland shocked them all. We played magnificently. It was a wonderful feeling leaving Pontypool Park being applauded off the field by a huge crowd of home supporters.

I think most doctors enjoy sport of one kind or another.

Medicine can be sad at times. We all need somewhere to escape, to get away from it all. Dr Hugh Philipps, from Llanboidy, was another sportsman in his day. He also did locum work to a good age, and he is remembered for some fine dentistry, too. That is how it used to be. Doctors did a bit of everything. Then it all changed. Of course, George tried to resist change, so Dolycwrt was still perfect for him – no computers, no appointments, but sadly no time off either. It was a bold stance to make, but I know he was determined about this. Malcolm and I wished him all the very best.

At this time of change, some of the Dolycwrt staff moved across to the new surgery. Over the years the doctors had been fortunate with their supporting team of nurses and receptionists. By now Leila Phillips, Esme Williams, Meinir Griffiths (previously Richards) had also been employed, with midwife, Stella Griffiths, among many regular visitors to the surgery. Stella, a popular lady in the locality, remembers all three of the doctors well. She has fond memories of working in some of the remote areas of the practice, when the doctors were only a phone call away:

> I had a lot of fun in the old days with Dr Penn, Dr Holding and Dr Allen. We had some memorable moments: Dolycwrt also being a big attraction as an old surgery that had survived to the modern day.
>
> I can remember being out in the wilds, miles away from anywhere, sometimes late at night, and with no one around to give directions . . . then having to cross fields with my medical bags. I would be wondering to myself . . . why a home delivery? When I called the doctors, I knew I would soon have some help. These are the occasions that I will not forget.

I must admit, I was sad when the partnership broke up, and so were many people. It had lasted a long time, but Dr Penn was from the Old School. He liked Dolycwrt too much. He really didn't want to move with the times, and he could be a naughty boy, too! He dug his heals in. He knew that group practice was not for him, and I'm sure he was right.

When I retired a few years later, we all met up in an evening get-together in the Picton Country Club, Llanddowror. We had a nice meal and we all had a few funny stories to share. True to form, Dr Penn was late again, arriving with Peggy towards the end of our meal. We had a photograph together, as I was presented with a beautiful hand-painted china ornament. Whenever I see this photo, I am reminded of some wonderful times at Dolycwrt. We were all good pals.

The Country Surgeries

BECAUSE OF THE WIDE geographical area of the practice, it is likely that even Dr Creswick Williams held some form of surgery when he went to the more distant villages like Llanglydwen years ago. It is possible that he used someone's dining room, or parlour, or perhaps a quiet room on the station platform, where it was convenient for him and his patients to meet. It is for this same reason that the Bont pub, Llanglydwen, is remembered as being a meeting place for doctors and patients from earlier times.

Likewise, as mentioned in *A History of a West Wales Village – Llanfallteg*, Dr Owen had a regular surgery at Hope Cottage, situated near the old station. This was certainly no later than the 1930s, because Dr Owen died in 1937. These venues, typical early-day country surgeries, played a big part in delivering healthcare to patients in rural locations when transport was limited. Many years later in 1983, the time of the big medical changeover in Whitland, the country surgeries were well established across the practice, each with its own stories to tell. They were as follows:

Cambrian House, Clynderwen	Monday	11.15am
The Post Office, Glandŵr	Tuesday	11.15am
Penybont Inn, Llanglydwen	Wednesday	11.15am
Market Hall, Crymych	Thursday	11.15am
Brynawel, Hermon	Friday	11.15am
The Shop, Tegryn	Saturday	11.15am

Up until this landmark year, they represented Dolycwrt. Often held on business premises open to the public – such as a shop, post office or public house – these surgeries, no doubt, helped trade, too. Certainly, they were big events, bringing activity and life into the country scene, whilst being a welcome change of routine for the doctors. For Dr Penn, he could escape into different surroundings for a few hours, and he looked forward to something that his predecessor Dr Gibbin enjoyed so much, meeting local characters in the natural surroundings of their home areas. Sadly for Dr Penn, however, when the partnership with Dr Holding and Dr Allen ended, responsibility for these surgeries fell upon the new group practice. Besides making regular appearances at Crymych Community Health Centre, for Dr Penn these happy occasions were all over, and were dearly missed.

At the pretty setting of Glandŵr – only yards away from the little river bridge that marks the confluence of the Rivers Taf and Gafel, as well as the small brook, nant Elwyn – Sally Lewis has fond memories of arriving with her family in the 1960s to run a post office and shop. Soon it became an important meeting place for the doctors and patients, and this continued for many years. Sally explained:

> There was an electric fire in the doctor's room and this was lit early every Tuesday morning. I also lit an open fire in the waiting room at the same time. Nobody was allowed to wait in the hallway, in case the doctors were heard; so, our sitting-room became the waiting room. There was seating for twelve or thirteen, and a lot were standing, too. Sometimes, patients did their shopping while they were with us. We sold a bit of everything, it was a village store. As far as I remember, most people walked to surgery. One day somebody brought a big dog along, and it was enjoying

lying in front of the fire. 'Dogs are not allowed in here, sorry,' I said. So he left and never returned.

One woman used to bring a library book with her, and she would sit in front of the fire half an hour before surgery started every week. When, one day, she did not arrive, someone suggested that she may be ill. To miss a surgery, she had to be ill!

The doctors took all prescriptions down to Mr Hughes, the Whitland chemist. The district-nurse dropped the medicines off at our post office, and people collected them from me. Sometimes, I had to stay up late into the night, because I didn't want to leave medicines in the porch outside.

The doctors were called away from surgery many times with urgent calls, and when they wanted a cup of tea, they went into the kitchen and helped themselves. I remember Dr Penn visiting me at ten o'clock one Christmas Eve. He had forgotten to buy a few presents. He also came to see me after the surgeries had ended. He missed them, and so did I. They were the happiest days of my life.

Dolycwrt says
Goodbye to the Old Mart Ground

B Y T H E M I D - 1 9 8 0 S, Dolycwrt had lost its long-term neighbour, the livestock mart. This celebrated institution that had brought the sound of farmyard activities to within earshot of the little surgery since Dr Creswick Williams' days, had moved to a larger site half a mile away. Gone were the days when animals either leapt from the trains leading to this famous piece of ground, or were directed there along the country roads and lanes. Maelgwyn James, a local farmer, regularly walked his father's cattle from beyond Tavernspite, more than three miles away, but this was not a problem because animals had a milder temperament then. Life was more natural and less stressful for them, too. The hard working horses exerted a different presence on the farms from our modern, noisy machines. Peace and harmony prevailed: 'just what the doctor ordered.'

Maelgwyn remembers the buzz of the mart, often teeming with rain on dark cold wintry days as animals, farmers, auctioneers and onlookers crowded into the enclosures and cramped spaces. Merchants, who had travelled into Whitland from different directions, having taken shelter under a shop canopy, laid their produce onto a little table. 'Who'll give me a pound for this watch?' they would call out, as people crowded round. Meanwhile, one hundred yards up the road, patients were being examined by the doctor in the rather quieter atmosphere of Dolycwrt. Maelgwyn continues:

Nobody wrote out a cheque in the street. There was an unwritten law: you had to settle your accounts in a pub. Of course, this suited most people. Mart days were happy, sociable events, bursting with life. Everyone enjoyed themselves. Others came to see what was going on; sometimes the doctors joined us, too.

This all changed with the new site. It was far more orderly, but it lacked the intimate atmosphere of the old ground. I suppose the modern marts had totally outgrown the original location. The bigger trucks and cattle wagons flooded into the town, and there was no room to move.

David Davies of Lampeter Velfrey was often seen on his horse and cart on mart days. David, a former member of Whitland Male Voice Choir, who sang alongside Dr Allen, when they performed at concerts, also remembers visiting Dolycwrt to see Dr Gibbin. He noted that despite the doctor's demanding medical duties, Dr Gibbin still found time for some farming. He kept his own livestock and was often seen around town on mart days. Dr Gibbin was totally at home in these important country gatherings, enjoying the hustle and bustle while talking to farming patients.

For David, who also remembers Dr Penn keeping a few cattle and entering them in Christmas fat stock shows, the old mart days bring back happy memories of past characters. One of his favourites was a traveller of no fixed abode who used to draw the crowds wherever he started his dancing act with a broom handle. He was also a man who always had a few tricks up his sleeve. One of these he saved especially for the mart days:

During the old days of the 1930s, many of the farmers used to drive their horse and carts into the Yelverton Hotel courtyard, where the horses were taken into the stables for food and rest. When the farmers went over to the mart grounds, or even into the pubs, Jack, as he was commonly referred to, would wander into the stables with a pair of scissors, and he would snip away at the horse's mane, or tug-away at its tail. Horse's hair was used as a fine twine for making cushions for settees and chairs, and he would sell it locally for a few bob. But when the old boys returned to the stables, they were upset.

One of these farmers was a gentleman named Tom Phillips. He had a horse named Dick and he was so fond of Dick that he used to smooth its tail all the way from Lampeter Velfrey to Whitland. For Dick not to have a long tail going home was very sad for Tom.

Keeping the Home Fires Burning

THROUGHOUT HIS term at Dolycwrt, Dr Penn continued to respect an old value that Dr Gibbin had, in earlier times, virtually written into its constitution. Although merely an old custom, it was vitally important for bringing ballast to Dolycwrt's ship, steadying its roughest passages, breathing life and loving care into its consulting rooms, and bringing much-needed warmth into the building. All of this refers to the residential caretakers, who gave the surgery a homely atmosphere. Over the years, many played their part, and each person can be proud of his, or her, contribution to Dolycwrt's great history.

It was during the late 1940s that Dr Gibbin left his surgery home, where Dr Owen – and Dr Creswick Williams before him – had lived with his wife and housemaids. Dr Gibbin was excited about Hafodwen: a new residence, built to his exact personal tastes, and situated in a countrified location on the outskirts of Whitland. But before moving, it was important for him to find suitable caretakers for Dolycwrt. This ensured that visiting patients received a warm welcome, arguably a potent tonic in its own right. This made Dolycwrt stand out like a beacon, shining bright, in all weathers, day and night. Indeed, beyond the war years of blackout rule, it was rare to see Dolycwrt without the lights on.

Gwladys Jones, previously Gwladys Smith, explained that Dr Gibbin offered her mother, Nan Smith, a native of Dr Gibbin's beloved Login countryside, a home at Dolycwrt.

This was when her husband, P.C. Tom Smith, died and the family had to leave the Police House in North Road. Gwladys lived with her mother in Dolycwrt for many happy years:

> If my mother went out to do some shopping – and I was working with Mr Mathias, the draper, then – Dr Gibbin made sure that he stayed on the premises in case of need. If ever mother was late returning, she could expect to see Dr Gibbin waiting on the backdoor step. He would not go from there. I remained in Dolycwrt until I got married. They were happy times, and we enjoyed the garden that extended down to the river, often having picnics on the back lawn.

Mair Mathias and her late husband, Roy, were the next care-takers, moving in during the late 1950s. Roy, who collected milk from the farms throughout a long career, also cut the grass at Parc Dr Owen for many years, dutifully driving the old tractor across the vast open green spaces, until the playing area looked like Wembley itself. Mair explained:

> I remember the solid wooden-block flooring which extended from our back room, down the passageway into the entire Surgery area. It was a lot of floor to keep clean, so I bought a second-hand polisher from Fred Thomas, the barber in King Edward Street. It was a strong, heavy electrical machine, ideal for Dolycwrt. When I finished the polishing, I was always proud of the result. It was a beautiful floor.

Both Gwladys and Mair remember a precise hand-over, ensuring that the premises and the phone were always manned. This is how it was when Mair's family later moved out. Dr Malcolm Holding and his wife, Pearl, then arrived, staying during the early 1960s with their young family. Dr

Holding, a keen fisherman, enjoyed the river at the bottom of the garden, beyond Stanley Griffiths' allotments, where he once caught thirty trout in a day – and emptied the river!

The next caretakers were Leon and Margaret Thomas, whose son, Michael, joined the Royal Navy. They made their back room warm and cosy, especially when the little log fire burnt away merrily in the grate. Leon and Margaret were amongst the first people in Whitland to have a new colour television, and they enjoyed their surgery-home for years.

Lloyd and Mary Evans were the next incumbents, before moving to the new medical centre in North Road, sometime around 1983. Lloyd remembers some very happy, and often, busy times when patients called at Dolycwrt:

> We used to see people arriving at all hours and met many local characters. We had a lot of fun with the doctors, too.

Then came John Mansfield, another lorry driver at the milk factory, and his wife, Olivia, and family. George Blethyn, by now a driver for Jones of Login coaches, and Eilir, his wife, replaced them. George was a long-serving member of Whitland Male Voice Choir and Eilir taught piano lessons. No doubt, this talented duo brought the sound of music to Dolycwrt. Eilir was from Llwyncelyn, Llanfallteg, where, during the era of the Cardi Bach, the blast of the steam engine leaving the little station was heard from her home:

> I was very fond of Dolycwrt and there was always something for me to do there, like cleaning the windows, washing the small cellar room, or varnishing the fire places. I enjoyed answering the telephones and meeting people when they called to see Dr Penn. It was a wonderful little surgery.

I had noticed medicine advancing over the years since my childhood days. My grandfather was a conductor at Capel Mair, Llanfallteg. I was told that one day he was taken ill with a perforated appendix. Two doctors from Haverfordwest, another from Narberth, and a nurse from Tenby, came out to Llwyncelyn and the operation took place on the kitchen table. This was in October 1914.

When George and I left, Myrddin John, his wife, Yvonne, and their young family replaced us. They stayed for a number of years, and they were the last of the caretakers during Dolycwrt's surgery days.

Dolycwrt escapes the Floods as Trevaughan Bridge lives on

S ITTING LOW IN the Taf valley, it is not surprising that Whitland has a history of flooding, but by the mid-1980s, these occurrences seemed to have run their course. However, following heavy rainfall in the late summer of 1986, the town felt the full force of a flood of great magnitude. Houses, shops, offices, pubs, the milk factory, and other buildings, such as the Senior Citizens Centre, took in serious amounts of water, as the town was turned into a sea of devastation. Many theories were suggested as to how this occurred, as major flood prevention work was carried out, without delay.

On this occasion, Dolycwrt was fortunate to be spared the commotion, seemingly standing on a little island surrounded by water, so it was business as usual the next day for the little surgery. Dr Penn had now adapted to life on his own, although well supported by his little team of Beryl Campbell and Anna Jones – Celia Leggatt, receptionist, and Nurse Eleanor Davies having both left by now – and Dolycwrt, which had tasted years of partnership medicine, was back as it once was in the days of Dr Creswick Williams. Dr Penn did not quite have the horse and cart, but he revelled in the traditional scene, enjoying country practice in his Morris Minor cars. He was now the owner of a new split-screen version, which he proudly added to his collection. Following years of commitment to Austin A35 cars, he was now pinning his faith on this favourite model of so many motoring enthusiasts.

Indeed, in a rapidly changing world, Dr Penn was now embracing as many of the old values and traditions as possible. Inside Dolycwrt, as well as outside, he clung to yesterday's standards, and he would not be swayed from this unconventional way of thinking. By this time, the late 1980s, most of Dr Penn's campaigning work had been done, but, when he then heard that Trevaughan Bridge was in danger of being demolished, he went along to see what he could do.

This famous old landmark, which had charmed Whitland's landscape for more years than people appreciated, was being replaced by a new structure. While the new roadway was welcomed and needed in the town, its arrival also meant that the town's little gem of a bridge was to disappear. While Dr Penn endorsed the concept of a new bridge, he was adamant that Whitland did not lose another piece of its precious stonework.

Attacking from all quarters, he asked Mr Rainbow, Whitland's photographer, to perform the task of taking photographs of the bridge and its beautiful archways. He then circulated these in his surgery waiting room and wherever he could, and arranged for water colours to be painted, too. The stone that depicted its age was a big find. Everyone soon realised that this really was an old treasure, rebuilt in 1767. In something of a compromise, the end of the bridge was removed, while the rest of it remained. It was not ideal, but the fight had been worthwhile. For Whitland, this was better than nothing.

At the Council Preservation Department, the officers kindly confirmed that this ancient structure is now listed as a 'good and substantial 18th century road bridge.' Indeed, it is far more than this; the beautiful stone pieces and cleverly crafted archways hold many secrets from the past. Besides witnessing the early doctors whose medical bags bulged with often unfriendly-looking instruments, they saw at first hand the night-time raids of the Rebecca Riots, when men on horseback attacked and destroyed the toll gates. In his book *The Rebecca Riots*,[59] Professor David Williams describes Whitland's part in these events during 1842 and 1843. At Trevaughan, the gate was situated beyond the bridge (when leaving Whitland) on the Pembrokeshire stretch of the river Taf, and, during these years, it was often destroyed.

The scene was now so totally different during Dr Penn's days, although he did give the people of Whitland a brief reminder of the old times when he jumped aboard a horse and cart for his second daughter's wedding in 1988. Dr Penn, accompanying Sarah to St Mary's Church, stopped on the bend of Trevaughan Bridge to be greeted by a large crowd of patients, friends and well-wishers, before he and Sarah proceeded to the church.

Most of Dr Penn's patients have treasured memories of this beautiful old bridge, and some of today's senior characters in the town smile about the days of their youth when one or two young and eager policemen, having just arrived, were tumbled over the wall for a cold and rather unpleasant bath. Nancy Williams who used to relieve the caretakers at Dolycwrt, shares some of her memories:

> I remember the old horse and carts crossing the bridge. We used to hear the clip clop of the hooves. The horses carried their heads high, proud animals, legs marching forward, wheels following behind. Then we heard 'Whoa boy!' as the cart drew to a halt. It was innocent, wonderful, and it is nice to look back on those times.
>
> Mr Richards, a farmer from outside Whitland, crossed the bridge most days. He would be taking the big round

---

59 Cardiff University of Wales Press, 1986

churns full of milk to the factory in his cart. I also remember Thomas and Morris, bakers, having an enclosed vehicle pulled by a horse. It made regular bread deliveries around Whitland.

In their day, all the doctors and nurses crossed the bridge and Dr Rowley Thomas was one of these. I once heard that he removed someone's tonsils on a kitchen table. We sometimes forget what the old doctors had to do.

At Dolycwrt, my brother, Leon, and his wife, Margaret – the surgery caretakers – used to keep Muscovy ducks at the bottom of the garden, alongside the river. Margaret used to have difficulties locating Dr Penn, and I can understand this, because I stayed in Dolycwrt to answer the phones when they visited their son, in Bermuda. Everyone wanted a part of Dr Penn, and he couldn't say no to anyone. I don't think he used a clock. He didn't know the meaning of time during work. And, he was driving an Austin A35, while Doctors Holding and Allen had faster cars.

Dr Penn often amused us at social functions with some of his tales. He once said he went to see a patient and told him to stay in bed until he called again. Three weeks later the man walked into the surgery asking if he could get up.

One of Dolycwrt's former patients, David (Dai) Skyrme recently departed the scene, shortly after celebrating his 70th year as a verger in St Mary's Church. David also received an agricultural award at the Royal Welsh Show for long service at Llwyndrissi farm, Whitland. It was during these farming years that David was called to help Dr Penn with his small-time 'farming' hobby. Although he had just the one field, Dr Penn enjoyed keeping cattle and rearing calves. Sometimes they would break through the fences, too, and David was always on hand to bring them safely back. He described a few memories of Trevaughan Bridge and the Dolycwrt doctors:

I remember the horse racing at Rhosgoch, when excited crowds crossed the bridge. Race meetings were keen events. One day, two local horses were in front on the final bend. There was a lot of shouting and cheering – because there was strong support for them both – and they crossed the line together. If there had been a camera that day, it would have been a photo-finish. But we had a man on the line instead. He had to pick a winner. His decision was final, but it was not popular. Many thought the wrong horse had the prize, and went home unhappy.

We would always see the doctors at the races. Dr Gibbin and Dr Evans would be enjoying themselves walking around, and talking to everyone. They were hoping for a quiet afternoon. They didn't want to treat patients at the races. All they wanted was for the jockey to stay on the horse's back.

When I was a child, we used to race along the top of Trevaughan Bridge. One boy would be on one wall, and another boy on the opposite wall. Then the rest of us would declare the winner. We all knew that if either had fallen, it would be a steep drop into the river – and we'd be running down the road to Dolycwrt. But this never happened.

Traditional Medicine sees
Dr Penn hitting the Headlines

THE WORLD had become so thoroughly modern by the time Dolycwrt entered into its last decade of medicine. Computers, mobile phones and gadgets had arrived, and the internet explosion was soon to follow, as the new hi-tech era swept aside all before it. For Dr Penn – positively resisting these new changes whilst upholding the traditional medical values of old – it could not have been easy. Yet he found it all immensely enjoyable.

Whilst he recognised the drawbacks of single-handed surgeries and the giant strides that had taken place to develop group practices, he was happy where he was. He would not consider stepping into the fast medical lane, preferring, what was for him, a more meaningful and quieter existence in Dolycwrt. Dr Penn was rooted to the old ways, and he would not change, regardless of the disadvantages.

Fundholding, targets and clinics, all favoured the group practices, as did the financial rewards, too. But, Dr Penn welcomed the freedom of serving patients fully, in his own time, in his own way, well supported by his staff and district nurses, such as Julie Phillips at this stage. He relished the moments, when, during quieter spells, he could visit his patients when they were fit and healthy. He enjoyed the social involvement that his privileged position allowed, and he could not envisage the end of these special days. He would soldier on in the old way with no computers, no appointment system and with a reliable Morris Minor car. He had cut through the woodland and trees into a land of freedom; he was enjoying himself.

Not so far away, in the Carmarthenshire fishing village of Ferryside, another doctor was upholding similar values and attitudes. No doubt, there were many more across the country, but they were becoming old-fashioned in more ways than one. Indeed, the systems in place ensured this. Dr Graham Jenkins was to Ferryside what Dr Penn was to Whitland: a lover of healing, close patient contact, paper files, and constant follow-up calls. He didn't favour appointment systems, and he would readily pick up his bag, day and night, to go to the place of his calling.

Ferryside is a delightful and picturesque village which blossoms into full colour in the beautiful, warm, sunny days of spring. It is for this reason that earlier in the century Whitland's church and chapel Sunday schools often chose Ferryside as the venue for their annual summer outings. Of course, it was easy to reach, because the railway took passengers to the heart of the village, just like it takes people into the main street of Whitland.

Dr Jenkins' son, David, also a doctor, told me that all the new systems and regulations saddened his late father by tending to get in the way of work as he used to enjoy it. Like Dr Penn, the late Dr Jenkins had considered medicine to be a recreation, enabling him to enjoy long dedicated hours, mixed with a little pleasure. David mentioned a follow-up call that his father made in Carmarthen one summer's day, when he set his boat free from its moorings, and sailed up the estuary. No doubt, his patient appreciated this, and Dr Penn would also have been impressed.

By the summer of 1992, Dr Penn's traditional ways of medicine at Dolycwrt were hitting the headlines. In the

Doctor magazine, on June 18th, shortly before Dr Penn's 65th birthday, a full-page feature described his unconventional approach. The heading boldly read 'G.P. takes to the hills to plough lone furrow.'

The article described the scene at Dolycwrt: the facilities, patients and Dr Penn's rather indifferent attitude towards retirement. Talking about his 24-hour-a-day commitment, and explaining that he preferred not to be included in a rota with his previous partners, Dr Penn admitted that patients even preferred the larger group practices. However, he felt the need for smaller concerns, too, believing that there was certainly a place for two-handed practices. The interview touched upon some of Dr Penn's earlier home confinements in the Dolycwrt Practice:

> once in the open air inside a circle of hippies strumming the guitar and humming, and once in a caravan besides a disused railway track and the River Taf.

Challenging the modern ways and concepts, Dr Penn described computers as 'a nine-year wonder' believing that people would want to revert to the old ways. Then, on the all-important subject relating to the continuance of Dolycwrt Surgery, he revealed his innermost thoughts and concerns:

> The key to whether it is taken over or not lies in the size of the practice and the quality of service. If these deteriorated the Family Health Service Authority would consider encouraging a merger with other practices.

Retirement Looms

B Y THE END OF 1994 the town of Whitland was still reeling from the unexpected closure of its proud milk factory. Having flown the flag of the Unigate Dairies and other concerns for many years – and later the bright colours of Dairy Crest – this source of huge employment for most of the century had sadly come to an end. It was an unbelievable situation that took everyone totally by surprise. There was no wind-down here; the factory gates were suddenly shut. It was a case of a working machine cut off in full swing, a giant chopped down in its prime. The bright lights of industry were turned into a still and total darkness overnight, seemingly, by the flick of a switch.

Next door, Dolycwrt continued to run its natural course of traditional medicine. It was too late to change now, but in a modern new world many people wondered how long it would last. The oil lamps that had once burnt so brightly in the consulting rooms had, long ago, gone out. Dolycwrt was equally susceptible to the same flick of a switch, especially as the new Health Centre was now established just up the road.

A year later, by the end of 1995, Dr Penn had secured the services of an assistant, Dr Frances Edwards, a lady doctor who had previously worked at Llanelli Hospital. He found her a great help, but, as is often the case, she was wanted elsewhere. She had received invitations from doctors in New Zealand; soon she would be going. For this reason, Dr Penn decided to look for another doctor straightaway. He considered that if someone stayed for a full year, then that person would have a chance of being able to stay permanently, even though this could not be taken for granted.

Through the contacts of a patient, Dr Penn had heard that a good doctor who had previously carried out considerable medical duties in Germany, and who was at the time doing general medical work for a Government Department, was interested in coming to Whitland.[60] This was Dr Ian Hood, a very qualified medical man, with a lot of hospital experience, too. Dr Hood started at Dolycwrt around May-time 1996 and, for a month, Dr Penn was in the unusual situation of having two assistants, with Dr Frances Edwards leaving for New Zealand the following month.

Dr Penn welcomed Dr Hood with open arms. He was able to personally introduce him to many of the patients, just as he had done with Dr Holding and Dr Allen in previous years. From that very beginning, he had hoped that there would eventually be permanence for Dr Hood at Dolycwrt, and everything was geared towards this. In the autumn of 1996, only eight months from Dr Penn's retirement date, he considered the time was right to make his last serious campaign.

In a long letter, dated September 26th 1996, to 'Patients and Friends of the Dolycwrt Practice' he explained that he was retiring and thanked everyone for their support. At the outset, he reminded everyone why he did not want to leave Dolycwrt in 1983 and set out the situation as it now stood with retirement looming. An extract appeared as follows:

> I now have an assistant doctor, Dr Ian Hood, with whom
> I am very well pleased and who likes the Practice and the
> whole area; in fact, he would very much like to stay after

---

60 Dr Penn's papers and records.

my retirement in May 1997, and I very much hope that this will happen.

However, there are difficulties in the way. With the increase in the number of doctors in Meddygfa Taf, the Dyfed-Powys Health Authority considers that there are probably enough doctors in the area already; so, at present, it is considered that I can't be allowed to make Dr Hood a partner, because that would mean adding an extra doctor to the list of doctors in Whitland.

In fact the Dyfed-Powys Health Authority in Carmarthen and the Medical Practices Committee in London have to decide whether or not the Dolycwrt Practice should be allowed to continue after my retirement. My number of patients being approximately 1,430 also raises doubts. If the number were as low as 1,000 the practice would probably be dispersed, but if the number was 2,000 the practice would probably be allowed to continue.

So, the first decision that has to be made is whether or not the Practice should continue. If it is allowed to continue, the Practice vacancy has to be advertised; Dr Hood could, of course, apply for it and he could be successful.

Then came his plea, perfectly wrapped, indeed disguised. It was the familiar call to duty, delivered in the usual soft manner, but, as usual, highly effective:

If the decision is made that the Practice can't continue, then Dolycwrt will have to go and patients will have to join another Practice. Many of our patients have already written letters appealing for the retention of the Practice and for Dr Hood to be allowed to take the Practice over. I do sincerely thank those who have already written; and I invite all who have not written to do so if they wish.

Letters should be sent to: Mrs Pat Archer-Jones, Director of Contractor Services, Dyfed-Powys Health Authority, Francis Well, Carmarthen.

To reaffirm his message, as seasoned campaigners do well, Dr Penn gently slipped in the next two sentences for commitment:

The letter need only be a simple plea to keep the Practice, or any other comments could be included if desired.

I believe that the Dyfed-Powys Health Authority might be influenced in their thinking by the many expressions of support for the Practice.

Dr Penn finished the letter with his usual pleasantries. Now he had thrown down the gauntlet for one last challenge, which continued for several months. Hundreds of patients wrote to the Health Authority, whilst support was sought from the Medical Committee, the Community Health Council, the local Community Council, and Nick Ainger, the local Member of Parliament.[61] The letter paved the way for success, but if there was any opposition to Dr Penn's motion at this stage, it was quickly swept aside by a tidal wave of good fortune:

As part of the campaign, one of our patients got the BBC Wales television people interested, and a team came to Dolycwrt one day. We appeared on the Welsh News, and also on the Welsh language TV and I think it made quite an impact. That is why they came back asking if they could film us in more detail in order to make a feature film as part of a series on the National Health Service. It has all been very exciting, and I was thrilled about that film. The

---

61 Dr Penn's papers and records.

BBC people cleverly picked up the threads of the whole situation, how we were campaigning to keep the Practice going, and for Dr Hood to take over, and I thought they brought it all into the film really well.

An Unforgettable Farewell

IN THE QUIETER days of October 1896 – a full century earlier and just two years before Dr Creswick Williams acquired the Dolycwrt premises – Mrs Wortley of the Waungron Estate in Whitland had invited her loyal tenants to a farewell dinner at the Yelverton Hotel. She was the widow of the late Major Wortley, who had been a director of the Great Western Railway. It was a very touching occasion, because she had sold the Waungron premises a little earlier. She looked back on a long period of happy relationships with her tenants. Now she was bidding them farewell, and had arranged for a chairman to read out her words. *The Welshman,* of October 30th 1896, reported. Below is an extract:

> I am truly sorry to part with each one of you as tenants … May I express a hope that the memory of 'the dear old master,' as you affectionately called my beloved husband, will be kept alive in the hearts of all present. I know you loved him; carry that love to your graves.

No doubt, this was a memorable event for all who attended. Yet, it was a sad ending to happier days. Now the clock was ticking away towards 16th May 1997, when Dolycwrt's medical baton would be passed over for the last time. It would be another unforgettable farewell.

After 42 years of service at Dolycwrt, Dr Penn was in need of a rest. Indeed, he had a heart complaint now that had aged him. However, this did not diminish his enthusiasm or excitement as his working days drew to a close. The public meetings in the town and the campaigning work were now finished. The panel representing the Dolycwrt patients – including Ray Vaughan, a close friend of Dolycwrt, who lived almost next door – had recommended a successor to the medical authorities. Everyone was happy with the nominee, Dr Hood. He had fitted in well in the community; he was the people's choice.

Following each step of the way during the last few weeks was Samantha Rosie and her BBC film crew. They were enjoying themselves away from Cardiff in the middle of the countryside, with all the local characters and their involvements. They were absorbed by the local events, taking every opportunity to gather more precious footage. On one occasion, Dr Penn's family were filmed having lunch. Whilst this did not make 'the cut,' it indicated how thorough their approach was. With Samantha looking through the lens of the camera, seeing everything at first hand, she is the best person to tell the story as the final day approached:

I remember arriving in Whitland. It was early spring time and Whitland seemed such a pretty place. Living in a world where purpose-built surgeries were now delivering medicine across the country, Dolycwrt was like walking back in time. I remember the beautiful stone frontage, and the gleaming brass name plate. I stepped into the passageway, onto the old floor tiling, and glanced to my right. There was Dr Penn's consulting room. I saw the fireplace, where a tall glass cabinet had been built into the wall on either side of it full of books, bottles, medicines, and tablets. I could only imagine how many consultations had taken place there over the years.

Near the window, there was a solid wooden desk full of

medical files, papers, prescription pads and diaries. There was an old eye chart on the wall, and also a patient's couch. There was a real atmosphere: this was a medical scene from the past, cosy and intimate. What a welcoming scene, so friendly and homely. I remember thinking . . . Wow, this is where patients had poured out their hearts to the doctors over the years; this is where generations of medical care had been delivered. I knew immediately that we had a story to tell. Dolycwrt had all the old values. Then Dr Penn appeared, smiling; I could see that he was proud of his surgery. To deliver such traditional medical ideals, there could be no greater champion than Dr Penn.

Of course, Dr Penn knew everything about his patients; he had delivered many into the world. He knew everyone's family connections vividly. He recognised when something was wrong: when people were, as he used to say 'off colour.' If something puzzled him, he would call at different times of the day to establish a pattern of symptoms, until he knew what was wrong. And he loved Dolycwrt. He wanted to see it continue as a surgery. He endorsed Dr Hood's intentions to succeed him; this was welcomed by the people of Whitland.

They were genuinely fond of Dr Hood. They had got to know him when Dr Penn secured him as an assistant. He wanted to carry on in the same vein, perhaps introducing a few modern inventions into the mix, like gadgets, computers, and more modern apparatus. But the local Health Authorities had their own agenda: they had to advertise the post. There was a real conflict, full of public participation; key characters with appeal; and an underlying outcome that was quite dramatic, quite final. And the stage was perfect – Dolycwrt – in the middle of lovely countryside. Screening this production was a joy.

We were documenting the changes in 50 years of the N.H.S. We were also capturing a moment of history in Whitland. There was no acting, there were no celebrities; this was a true story.

We went everywhere with Dr Penn. We were in his Morris Minor; I loved that car. Together we experienced the Comet Eclipse; this was happening at the time. Dr Penn was so immensely humble. I remember a farmer coming into the surgery with a mole. Dr Penn loved to get the silverware out; he was so proud of his minor operations. On another occasion, we visited Sir Eric Howells, before travelling to see a patient in the country. Dr Penn was so perfectly natural with them both. Dr Penn enjoyed looking after the holidaymakers at Pendine. This is where we filmed the closing scene, as he walked along the beach, alone. The sun was setting. It was very touching.

Everyone in the practice recognised the part that Dr Penn's wife, Peggy, played in Dr Penn's story. She was wonderful. Peggy used to answer the phone, and kept the home fires burning, allowing Dr Penn freedom to do his work in his inimitable way. We went up the drive and saw this magnificent white residence with a porch entrance. There were lovely lawns and trees all around with stunning views. Around the back, I remember Dr Penn's old cars. He had quite a collection. Then we stepped into the vegetable garden, so peaceful, so private. Beyond it was the orchard, another world.

When we returned to the BBC, our problem was to edit hours of quality footage into a 30 minute show. I was thrilled when we produced an award-winning documentary. It was the perfect tribute to Dr Penn's wonderful career. All these years later, I am still reminded that this was my best production. We called it *The Doctor's Story*.[62]

Samantha was there on the last day, May 16th 1997, the day before Dr Penn's 70th birthday. It was one of those action-packed occasions, with patients, friends, nurses, and well-wishers calling with gifts, cards, presents, cakes, messages and gestures. It was all very touching: very special – exhausting, too. Dr Hood was there and Dr Penn's little team: Beryl Campbell, practice nurse, and receptionists, Elizabeth White and Rhys Adams. They would experience changes now. This was the end of an era.

The local papers had reported all events of the past few weeks, indeed months. It had been a media bonanza. Dr Penn was a celebrity. Headlines, such as, 'Fight on to save Whitland surgery,' 'Patients join the bid to save doctor's practice,' and 'Doc hangs up his stethoscope,' appeared in the local newspapers. There would be parties to follow, and much more news coverage, too, and the goodbyes were far from finished, but here was the moment of truth. It was mid afternoon, the camera team was poised to take one last shot: Dr Penn being invited outside. Retirement awaited – no more patients, or problems, or medicines, or minor operations.

He emerged from the little operating room, which Dr Gibbin had built as a small extension for his dispensary, probably around the 1950s. This room hid the old side door where patients in previous times would knock and wait. There Dr Owen or Dr Creswick Williams, or their wives or maids, would answer. That little recess could tell a tale or two, but for years it had been a cupboard, where Dr Penn kept some of

---

62 The BBC's *Tales from the Health Service*, a series of documentaries, celebrating the 50th Anniversary of the birth of the National Health Service.

his surgical instruments. He made his way towards the little doorway for the last time.

Dr Penn was not alone; he never was alone. His wife, Peggy, was always there for him, and she would be sharing this special moment, too. In some ways she had lost out to medicine and the railways and campaigns and Whitland Weeks, but this did not worry her. She would be there to welcome him home whatever the time of day or night. She was proud to. From the days of Neath General Hospital in the early 1950s when she called out, 'Calling Dr Penn. Dr Penn, you're wanted at reception, please,' she had been his best friend. She had waited 18 months for him to return from Nigeria and had followed him ever since; she wanted nothing more. Peggy was private; Dr Penn was public. Together they were quite a team.

Without them knowing, the school children and teachers had quietly filed into the garden. The front lawn was a sea of faces, mostly the little faces of children, but there were others, too. This was an impressive site: the stage was set; it was time for 'Action please!' And out they went – Dr Penn first, Peggy following by his side. On the step they stopped momentarily, before Dr Penn walked forward a few paces. He faced the cameras, the children, and the entire school.

It was the same little school which Dr Creswick Williams closed during epidemics of scarlet fever and measles way back in Queen Victoria's days; it was the same little school that stood in ceremony when Dr Owen's funeral cortège left for Soar Chapel in 1937; it was the same little school that Doctors Gibbin, Evans, Penn, Holding and Allen had served in their time whilst probably presenting prizes on sports days, as was the early custom. Indeed, it was the same little school, like a neighbour – no, like a big brother – that was there before Dolycwrt, and saw it grow, and would be there after it, too.

The children had arrived with their placards. One of these, everyone's favourite, simply read, 'Dr Penn – too young to retire.' They were ready to sing as well; a delightful mixed junior choir bursting into 'Pen-blwydd Hapus' (Happy Birthday in Welsh).

Then little Craig Storer of Whitland stepped forward with a gift of flowers. It was his job to make a presentation; indeed, he made an impact, too.

'Thank you, Craig; thank you very much,' said Dr Penn.

'Thank you, Dr Penn . . .' replied Craig, 'for saving my life!'

Dr Penn was never short of a word or two: his eloquence was manifest in all he did. But on this occasion, he had to dig deep, but out they came, every word carefully chosen, at this most poignant moment in the day.

Smiling, facing Craig, facing everyone, and facing retirement, he replied,

'I'm really overwhelmed. It's terrific; most beautiful; most wonderful; most memorable; most unforgettable.'

A Remarkable Century

IN THE DAYS THAT followed, Dolycwrt reverted to what it knew best and became a surgery once again. The excitement had died down. It was no longer a film studio, or meeting place, or party venue, and the caretakers, Myrddin and Yvonne John, and their family, could also live normal lives again. As usual, there were patients to see, and the rigours and demands of modern medicine were many, especially from the confines of a sole practitioner's seat. It could not have been easy for Dr Hood, and who could envy him taking over the challenging grip of Dolycwrt's reins? Yet, Dr Hood made a big impression. He cared for the local people and was well liked. He, too, was carving his initials in the Dolycwrt walls, and people wished him well.

As much as Dr Penn was enjoying a quieter life, he was still living in the land of celebrities, enjoying this, too. He loved being surrounded by people. At his home, he welcomed everyone who called by, happily sitting and talking on the lawns. The letters, cards, poems, messages and gifts had slowed down, although they continued to trickle through for quite some time. He was now working on a speech. Dr Penn was always known for his long speeches; this one would be longer than most. He had arranged an evening dinner at Nant-y-Ffin Motel, to celebrate his retirement. He had invited a large number of medical people, including consultants from the local hospitals, as well as friends.

There, he talked about his life and medical years. He

spoke about his time with Dr Gibbin and how he settled into the town in 1955. He thanked Dr Holding and Dr Allen and the consultants, and everyone, for the help that he deeply appreciated. He mentioned the last few years of his career in Dolycwrt, when he enjoyed being the official doctor for the Bourne Leisure Pendine Holiday Caravan Village. 'There I enjoyed meeting so many of the happy people on holiday,' he mentioned. Indeed, Pendine brought variety to his daily routines, refreshing, just like the sea air. He praised the work of Kaye Davies, proprietor of a large local haulage company. 'I have also enjoyed being the doctor of Mansel Davies and Son Limited, Llanfyrnach. What a happy outfit I consider that to be.' Then, regarding his years of campaigning, he had a funny story to tell.

It was back in the 1960s, and he was fighting to save the Tenby railway line. He had invited the BBC radio crew to witness a large gathering of people boarding the train at Whitland. 'It all went well,' he said, 'except for one Whitland gentleman who, when asked by the BBC radio reporters why the train was so full that day, replied that he had no idea – that he couldn't make it out – that normally there were only two or three in the town. I could have crowned him!'

There then followed a special evening in the Whitland Town Hall in the warm summer of June 1997. This same landmark building had locked away, within its tall walls, the secrets of Whitland's social events since 1904. Now, the newly renovated Hall was looking resplendent for a very different event. As a large crowd settled down inside, Whitland's talented Peter Wills was preparing back stage. He was wearing his Eamonn Andrews suit now, and the famous Red Book was in his hands. Soon he would be saying, 'Tonight, Dr Penn: This is Your Life!'

Tracing Dr Penn's life back to his birth in 1927, many

events from his colourful past unfolded. Among those attending were the Mayor of Whitland, Bill Allen; Dolycwrt practice nurse, Mrs Beryl Campbell; Dr Penn's successor, Dr Hood, as well as consultants from both Withybush and Glangwili Hospitals. Mr Russell Davies, a farmer from Efailwen, took to the stage. He thanked Dr Penn for treating him during the snow expedition with the helicopter, back in 1982. And there were many more surprises in a thoroughly entertaining evening, which ended with a magnificent buffet. This show had been a well-kept secret for months and, besides Peter Wills, many others had been busy organising it. For Dr Penn, it was a total shock; he thought he was going to a concert.

If Dr Penn believed that his high-profile departure would end here, he was wrong. On September 27th that same year, 1997, Samantha Rosie's documentary appeared on BBC Wales; it was a major success. But, when it was later shown to the British nation on BBC Two, it prompted national newspaper reviews, such as the *Daily Telegraph's* headline 'It shouldn't happen to a doctor' – as well as letters from friends and colleagues. Below is a message sent by a former sole practitioner:

Dear Dr Penn,
Last night I sat with tears in my eyes watching the T.V. programme about you and your practice.

I am a G.P. of your generation, and I started work in a rural practice. I had the same ideals and, I hope, the same dedication as you, but over the years the practice grew to eight partners – and it was not possible to continue to practice the same sort of medicine which I had always done. After 30 years in the practice, I reluctantly left . . .

There was another letter, too, highlighting the golden times of general practice which Dolycwrt had facilitated throughout the years. A brief extract reads:

Dear George,
What a wonderful programme and what a tribute to you for the sincerity you brought to your work over all those years. I have always known the regard in which Uncle Dick was held; now I realise that you are of the same school.
I do congratulate you and wish you and Peggy well.
Very sincerely,
Jo

This was from the late Jo Morris, Dr Owen's niece. She left one last message at the foot of the letter:

The programme missed one very important fact – Dolycwrt is where I was born in 1924.

The next year, 1998, marked a full and rounded century of medical years at Dolycwrt. Since its start date on 10th November 1898, during times of the horse and cart, it had progressed to the days when man walked around on the moon. The last locum, Dr Frances Edwards, had quietly left Dolycwrt to start another job in New Zealand, the other side of the world. Dolycwrt's journey in time had been extraordinary, to say the least. Along the way, medicine had changed greatly; indeed Dr Penn was now sporting another recent invention – a heart regulator, known as a pace-maker. There would be no end to medical advancements now. General Practice was different, too, the odds being firmly stacked against the single-handed practitioner. When work systems are redesigned to change the future, things either fall into line, or fall out of favour. It is as simple as that.

These thoughts reminded me of the words I heard at St Mary's Church from Reverend Kingsley Taylor. He had just returned from an earlier service at Llandissilio, and he was captivated by the beautiful show of greenery as he travelled down Pengawse Hill into the Taf valley.

'Isn't it wonderful,' he asked, 'how nature always knows what it is trying to do? Only a few months ago, we were in the grip of freezing ice and snow. But now, here we are in spring, with everything turning to green.'

He related this to human limitations, and how we were powerless to such perfection.

'And why?' he asked, turning to the congregation. 'Well, it's simply because we are living in a world that is bigger than us.'

This simple, but highly effective, statement can be related to Dolycwrt. Despite having been a doctor's surgery for 100 years, it was now swimming against the tide. Why? Well, because Dolycwrt was standing alongside bigger local Group Practices where there were clinics, modern facilities, more staff and considerable economies of scale. It was living in a world that was bigger than itself. It had survived a full century. As regards more, perhaps it was not meant to happen.

As it transpired, Dr Hood left his post later in the year, for personal reasons. Again this prompted more campaign work to keep the surgery open, but this was never going to materialise. Dr Penn was deeply saddened, knowing that there would be no favourable result – not this time. The previous reprieve had given Dolycwrt the chance that everyone fought for. There would be no other. Time had marched on again; in fairness to the Health Authorities, they had already honoured their side of the bargain.

In 1871, in the South Kensington region of London, looking onto Hyde Park, a very special building was completed, that still stands head and shoulders above the rest. It is an old treasure from yesterday. From the outside it appears like a rounded dome full of windows, letting in daylight into its secret inner sanctums. Inside, the rows of terraced galleries; and towering pillars; and royal-red coloured seats; and high ceiling, elevate it in a striking manner to the status of a 'theatre of dreams.' But the Royal Albert Hall is more than that. The Royal Box adds the important seal of Royal approval, and this is where Queen Victoria ventured in her horse-drawn carriage – before either our school or surgery ever existed – for its official opening.

Every year this famous, fabulous setting opens its doors to the Henry Wood Promenade Concerts. For those lucky enough to experience the 'last night' they participate in a free flowing, carnival-like atmosphere of fun, flags, laughter and lots of community-like singing. Every year, the grand finalé is the singing of *Land of Hope and Glory*, when everyone readily and merrily bursts into song, raising the high roof further into the London sky.

Every year also, the Royal Albert Hall hosts the Royal British Legion Festival of Remembrance Service. This year it was staged on Saturday 7th November 1998, exactly three days short of a full one hundred years since Dr Creswick Williams took ownership of the Surgery. This is a very different service. It is stately and sober, structured by years of traditions and precedents. There, our proud men and women of Her Majesty's Forces march onto the floor immaculately regaled in their smart uniforms. Next come the Veterans, our much older war heroes, decorated with their gleaming medals. And so it continues one scene after another, wave after wave of colour, military discipline and decorum, during a night to honour our fallen heroes.

That year, sitting in seats one and two, of Box 22, on the

second tier, was the longest serving of the Dolycwrt doctors. Dr and Mrs Penn had always wanted to attend this service and, in recognition of their past British Legion work, they had been rewarded. They were excited and honoured, and had arranged for their gardener, David Jones, to take them by car. David had himself served in the Forces, and getting Dr and Mrs Penn to the front door of the Royal Albert Hall, in the busy London traffic, was itself a military exercise. The service was a stirring occasion that lived on in their memories with a great sense of pride.

Who could forget that magnificent arena where Wagner, Verdi, Elgar and Rachmaninov had performed? where Her Majesty the Queen and Sir Winston Churchill and Bill Clinton had spoken? and where Frank Sinatra and the Beatles had entertained? Dr and Mrs Penn certainly would not. They were sitting in anticipation, soon to be enthralled. Peering down, listening out – but also looking back. Yes, it was hard not to. Dr Hood's departure had been a terrific blow; it was a shock that hit Dr Penn hard. While the Surgery doors would remain open until the early months of the new year, he knew that its end had already arrived. In real terms, it was all over. He was not wrong. Glancing at his programme, he would have noticed two lines of that most treasured favourite, *Abide with Me*. Those few words would say so much:

> Swift to its close ebbs out life's little day;
> Earth's joys grow dim, its glories pass away.

In every corner of the world, things are coming to an end every day. Indeed, this most resplendent, this most regal, of occasions was also coming to an end. Undeniably, this has been the theme of this story throughout: beginnings and endings, doctors coming and doctors going. Dr Penn had never mentioned Dr Creswick Williams because he didn't know him like we do; yet Dr Penn knew someone had held high the medical lantern of his proud profession during those dark days. Of course, he had heard of Dr Owen's great qualities, and he had stood alongside Dr Gibbin as his junior partner. They had all come and gone, having carried Dolycwrt's medical mantle – just as he and Dr Hood had done – into a new era. As for the fortunes of the little surgery, these lay in the first line of the last hymn that night:

> The day thou gavest, Lord, is ended,
> The darkness falls at Thy behest.

Every man and every woman took a deep breath, as the last verse fell upon them. In the days of Queen Victoria and her succeeding monarchs, people outside this wonderful building would have heard the rousing singing of music festivals long before even the Great War. Since television had arrived in the 1950s, every scene and every word of this Remembrance Service entered the homes of millions of people. Soon, it was time to raise that roof again, to fill the magnificent arena with the beautiful and powerful and sad words, of this cherished hymn:

> So be it Lord; Thy Throne shall never,
> Like earth's proud empires, pass away;
> Thy kingdom stands, and grows for ever,
> Till all thy creatures own they sway.

Soon the bugler would be heard: what an honour for that person; what a proud history is associated with this – the *Last Post*. Then, that most poignant of all moments: that chilling, humbling experience, when we can do nothing more than bow our heads in honour of our fallen heroes. This year, as the poppies fell in the Royal Albert Hall, the final curtain fell on Dolycwrt. Why we may ask, does everything come to an end? Well, we may know the answer now, or, at least, the vicar has given us a clue: 'It's simply because . . . we are living in a world that is bigger than us.'

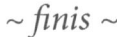

~ *finis* ~

ABOUT THE AUTHOR

ROGER PENN is the son of the late Dr George Penn and his wife, Peggy. He is a native of Whitland and attended the local primary and grammar Schools before joining Lloyds Bank Limited in 1976.

After a 34-year career, Roger retired in January 2010, still a believer in the traditional bank values of old. He served in many branches across south Wales between Newport (Pembrokeshire) and Chepstow, whilst also venturing into the Forest of Dean at Lydney, Gloucestershire, in 1982. His last post was in his father's hometown, Bridgend, at the Wyndham Street Branch.

Roger has an unswerving passion for Dolycwrt and its proud traditions and history. This is where he lives today with his wife, Celeste, enjoying the house and garden which date back to the days of the first doctor.

Known as 'Dr Penn's son' in his homeland, Roger is a rugby enthusiast, who for many years travelled extensively throughout the principality as a Welsh Rugby Union referee. Roger is a student of the written word, and is now dedicating more time to writing. He also enjoys contributing to community life in Whitland, and is particularly keen to see our treasured little towns and villages restored to their former glory.

Roger has a selection of small publications to his name, but this is his first major work.